Weight...
It Might Be Your
Thyroid

Weight… It Might Be your Thyroid – Dr. Michael Scott

Published in the United States by Cube17, Inc.

ISBN: 978-1-945196-02-7

www.drmichaelscott.com/

www.themilliondollarbookclub.com

TABLE OF CONTENTS

Introduction

Diabetes, obesity and other heart-related problems have long been a major threat in the US. Between the years 2008 and 2015 alone, obesity rates have dramatically increased by twenty-eight percent. In a nutshell, over the course of seven years, six million more adults have joined the long list of Americans who are suffering from obesity. In addition, over twenty-nine million Americans are diagnosed with diabetes, which ranks seventh in the top causes of death in the US, while eighty-six million more show pre-diabetic symptoms. With these statistics in mind, this book hopes to shed some light on the otherwise bleak future of American health.

There are countless diet programs out on the market, and each one claims to be the ultimate solution to the never-ending weight loss journey. However, many people are becoming more and more desperate and almost hopeless, due to having tried and tested every single diet trend but without any real and lasting effects. If you're one of these people, then this book might possibly be the answer to your problems.

Who Will Benefit from this Book?

This book is especially for those of you who are tired of yo-yo diets and rebound weight gain. I understand how you feel. A lot of people have experienced, and are still experiencing, the very same dilemma you experience. You go up and you gain weight and then you go down and you lose weight, up and down, then down and up like a yo-yo. The problem is that you follow all these programs without considering that perhaps you have an issue with your thyroid. You can starve yourself, you can go to the gym three times a day, but you're not going to lose weight. If your thyroid is not functioning the way it's supposed to, it doesn't matter what you do. Improve your thyroid, only then you will start seeing lasting results.

People of all ages can benefit from the safe and effective weight loss methods presented in this book. Whether you're fourteen or forty years old, you can lose weight and maintain it. They say that it is normal to be overweight after reaching forty years of age. I say, it isn't. If it were true, then everyone over forty in the entire world should be overweight. But that's not the case. That is a mere myth and a hundred percent false. You shouldn't let this common misconception seal your fate. You can take control of your body. All that is needed is a little science.

So What Sets It Apart from All Other Weight Loss Books You've Read?

First and foremost, it presents a scientific approach to your weight issues. Instead of offering what you call a Band-Aid solution to the severe and advanced weight problem, this book offers a deeper, more efficient and more lasting solution. In order to cure any disease, the very root cause, and not just the superficial symptoms, should be addressed. Curing the symptoms alone may give temporary relief, but will not have a lasting effect. In other words, you shouldn't trim weeds. It will make your garden look neat and nice for a little while, but it will grow back in just a matter of time. In order to maintain your garden, what you need to do is to pull the weeds from their roots.

This book is meant to educate the readers about the significance of the thyroid gland in losing and maintaining weight. In short, we offer a healthier, more substantial weight loss strategy for you and your loved ones. Losing weight is not just about looking good; more importantly, it's about feeling great and being able to function to your full potential. Thus, you should take care of your body and lose weight the healthy way. There's no actual need to starve yourself and deprive your body of its basic needs in order to look good. On a deeper note, you should lose weight in order to boost your health, immunity and longevity, which are imperative in achieving happiness, meaning and purpose in life.

What Will You Get After Reading This Book?

If you've tried all sorts of diets and signed up for expensive weight loss programs, but without getting the desired results, it might be because of your thyroid. Your thyroid plays a major role in your metabolism, and metabolism is a key factor in weight loss. Your thyroid hormones are responsible for hastening or slowing down your metabolism. Unfortunately, we're exposed to so many toxins from the food we eat, throwing our hormones out of balance, and negatively affecting our gut ecology. Most of us may not know it, but we might actually be suffering from a deficient thyroid system.

This book will teach you how to successfully and safely lose and maintain weight by changing certain patterns in your metabolism. Understand that metabolism is not static, but is subject to constant change. By improving this function, you are paving a clear and easy path to healthy weight loss. How can your metabolism improve? By taking into account your thyroid gland and regulating your thyroid hormones, which are factors responsible for good metabolism. You will learn how to correctly identify factors suggesting an issue with your thyroid, and address each one properly.

Another major thing in this book, which you will be very thankful for, is that you can still enjoy most of your favorite food without compromising your weight loss goals. Self-starvation and self-deprivation are not on our plate. We also do not promise instant weight loss. What we can promise is healthy and effective weight loss that will last. By following the suggestions in this book, you will slowly but surely lose weight. You will learn how to lose weight, and maintain healthy weight, not just for a couple of months down the road but for the rest of your life. All you need to do is incorporate some very easy lifestyle changes that won't necessarily push you far beyond your comfort zone.

After improving the health of your thyroid and restoring the proper hormonal balance in your body, you're on your way to achieving fitness, health and happiness.

Why I Wrote This Book

Well, the story begins with my childhood dream of becoming a doctor. I wanted to become a doctor for prestige and, of course, to make my parents proud. So I did my best in school and earned good grades, because I really wanted to go to medical school. But the real turning point in my young life was not in my academic efforts but in my athletic activities. I was a sprinter and also played defense on our school's football team. One morning, I woke up with a really bad back ache, perhaps due to an unattended injury which is quite unavoidable when you're into sports. I was taken to a chiropractor, and a couple of sessions later, my back pain was gone. That was my first experience with a chiropractor. As a matter of fact, that was also the very first time I'd ever heard of a chiropractor. Before that, I never knew that such a medical profession existed.

So, anyway, let's fast-forward to my time in medical school. Medicine being a symptom-based profession, I've seen patients being given a lot of medications for fixing symptoms, instead of finding out the root of the problem. But if you really come to think of it, with medication, the symptom may go away but the problem doesn't necessarily go away. And from the very beginning, this never felt okay with me. Perhaps my intuition pointed me back to the memory of how a chiropractor helped me with my back injury, by targeting the root problem in my spine and not simply by giving me painkillers. The experience really made an impression in me and, so, I decided to still carry on with my medical course, but this time focusing on chiropractic care.

However, after my first year in chiropractic school, I felt really limited. I found that the focus was basically on mechanical injuries and fixing the spine and some of the neurology as it relates to the spine. I felt like I needed to expand my knowledge, and so I started attending specialty courses on functional neurology in the Carrick Institute of Clinical Neuroscience while I was a student in chiropractic school. While studying functional neurology, I met a gentleman who told me about functional medicine, something I've never heard of before. He said that functional medicine is about actually finding the cause of a patient's symptoms and fixing the cause. And, at that point, it was a Eureka moment for me. Not wanting to do another 3 to 4 years of residency in med school, and wanting to have autonomy, I decided to finish my chiropractic schooling simultaneously with my functional neurology course. After that, I took a course on functional medicine.

So what inspired me to focus on the aspect of weight loss?

Here's the story. As part of our internship program, we had to see patients under the supervision of a licensed doctor. A thirty-nine-year-old patient by the name of Karla was assigned to me. She had a back issue, somewhere in her upper back near the shoulder area. Taking the patient's history, one thing that stood among the other typical symptoms of back pain was her twenty-pound weight gain in the last year. She didn't feel normal about it, but her doctor told her otherwise. He said that her test results were normal, since she was nearing forty. He said that at that age, metabolism slows down. But that was the first time I heard that theory, really.

She confided that she didn't feel it was normal at all. She was distraught. She had always been a slender, athletic person with great muscle mass, but she had gained a lot of fat. And she couldn't figure out why she kept on picking up weight, when she is by no means a sedentary person. After the unexplained weight gain, she went from being an outgoing and confident woman who loved hanging out with a lot of friends to a devastated, insecure person who felt less attractive and thus shied away from her usual activities. Her entire outlook in life changed. Her opening up and confiding in me was deeply moving. During that time as an intern, I hadn't seen that many patients before. And for the most part, they were simply mechanical. So this was a different experience, a very personal one. Something about her story moved me to want to help her. Perhaps I was able to relate to her because I was an athlete myself. I also regularly go to the gym and have never gained weight like she had.

I looked deeper into her medical records to see what type of testing had been done. Her TSH (Thyroid Stimulating Hormone) and T4 (the inactive thyroid hormone, which needs to be converted to T3) results were fine. But I did detect many markers that seemed important. Initially, I suspected that she had some sort of inflammation in her system that was keeping her from losing weight. But, then again, I was a newbie, an intern. I asked her to have her doctor run more tests, not knowing that most of the time, most doctors don't want to do it. Fortunately enough for Karla and for me, her particular doctor was open to running those tests. In addition to her TSH and T4 tests, we also tested for her T3 and reverse T3. Her reverse T3 was fine, but her T3 was extremely low. But let's save this specific and broad topic of thyroid hormones for another chapter. Moving on, I suggested that she start on a selenium supplement to help with the regulation and re-balancing of her hormone levels. Two weeks later, she was down six pounds just from this mineral. A Selenium supplement is taken in supplement form with water. As easy as that, you will not have to resort to starvation, surgery or other drastic measures just to obtain your target weight.

Amazingly, this minute correction in her body translated into a major correction in her weight, and an even bigger correction in her attitude and mental stability. Moreover, the advice was given by a mere intern. The point is that we need to understand that it's not rocket science. You don't have to be a genius to understand how your body works, how it can gain or lose weight. It's also not difficult to understand that weight loss or weight gain is a symptom of the cause, and not the problem itself.

To make my point clear, allow me to use an analogy. Take, for instance, that you have a defective car. You know there's something wrong with it somehow, but you use it anyway. So you end up immobile and stuck in the middle of traffic, and then ultimately get towed. Similarly, you know you've tried almost every diet program there is but without achieving the desired result. Still, you carry on and go on hopping from one diet program to another. In the end, you end up gaining even more weight, feeling more insecure, and losing a lot of money in the process. On the other hand, if you try to get at the root cause of your weight problem, instead of making superficial and often irrelevant changes, you will save yourself a lot of time, energy, money, stress and frustration.

Meeting Karla was the main turning point, in my life, that made me decide to focus on weight loss. I could never forget the look on her face when she came back two weeks later and thanked me for helping her lose weight. Gradually, she bid goodbye to her insecurities and went back to being her normal outgoing self.

At that point, I knew in my heart that this is what I wanted to do. I want to truly help people understand why they can't lose weight despite all efforts. In the majority of the patients I've dealt with, once their thyroid problems are fixed, they become better people. And it's very heartwarming and fulfilling to know that I am somehow being able to help people not just physically, but most importantly emotionally.

What does this book offer?

The main focus of this book is to help you properly identify the root cause of your weight gain, so we can fix it and subsequently eliminate the symptoms.

The dieting industry focuses on giving people some 'magical' weight loss pill, or a temporary fix of the symptom. We, on the other hand, apply functional medicine to weight loss. We will help you find out why you are overweight, instead of just giving you a pill to temporarily alleviate the symptoms.

Weight… It Might Be your Thyroid – Dr. Michael Scott

We will help you put the balance back in your hormones. Once the root cause is identified and given due attention then, as a result, the symptom of weight gain will be eliminated. You will be able to successfully lose fat weight, and not muscle weight or water weight. Let me share with you the harsh reality behind most diet programs.

In most of these weight loss programs, people are fed with false hope. They think they're losing weight, but in fact, they're only losing water weight or muscle weight, which is quite normal in the early phase of any weight loss program. You see, most of these programs promote calorie restriction, which also means restricting the amount of proteins and good fats. In this case, your body will innately start to rely on muscle for fuel and energy. That's the weight loss that you actually experience. You may be on a six-hundred-calorie diet for three months, and you may lose thirty pounds. The problem is, once you get back to your normal eating habits, your body will naturally want to gain back those muscles. Remember that muscle holds a little bit more weight than fat. Once you gain those muscles back, which you will in due time, you will undoubtedly gain back those pounds. You think the program works but it's just a trick, a sham. You lose a lot of weight in the first month but you don't lose any more in the succeeding months because there is no more muscle. Your metabolism is probably slowing down because you have less muscle. You may drop a few pounds, but in reality, you're getting sick. Here's what actually happens inside your body.

As you lose those muscles and as you restrict those calories, your body goes through a state of starvation. As a result, it starts holding on to as much fat as it can while slowing down its metabolism. By starving your body and depriving it of good fats and proteins, you're putting it in quite the opposite position. It's not going to be able to lose weight. It's simple science, really. This is just your body's coping mechanism when under the threat of starvation. Furthermore, nighty-five-percent of the time, after you stop restricting your calories, your body will naturally want to gain back the weight lost and restore your health. Since your body's metabolism has slowed down, you will gain back weight with a vengeance. It's like rebound weight gain. This is what you call the yo-yo pattern.

By relentlessly jumping from one diet program to another, you arc driving your body into sheer exhaustion. Starving yourself and then binge eating, and then starving yourself all over again and binge-eating again. It becomes an ugly habit, a nasty and destructive cycle that will damage your body in the long run. More significantly, you are damaging not only your physical health, but also your emotional and mental well-being. Multiple failures in losing weight can be frustrating, discouraging and shattering.

For most people, it would be easier to succumb to and accept being overweight and obese. But the goal of this book is to reach out to people who are almost on the point of giving up. You can lose weight successfully and safely. You simply have to admit that your body naturally knows what to do. Together, we can take away the barriers and let your body do its natural healing process. We offer to help you maintain the muscles and lose the extra fat that your body knows it doesn't need.

Why am I writing this book?

You, Karla and countless other people are my inspiration.

Your over weight, now what?

There are some inherent health risks for being overweight. The top 3 diseases associated with being overweight include:

High Blood Pressure. This is the most common problem with overweight people. Blood pressure is the force of blood being pushed against the walls of the arteries as the heart supplies blood to the body.

Coronary Heart Disease. CHD is a condition when there is a buildup of a waxy substance called plaque in the coronary arteries. The function of the arteries is to supply oxygen-rich blood to the heart. The buildup of plaque can block the coronary arteries and weaken the flow of blood to the heart muscles. This eventually leads to angina or chest pain and to what is commonly known as a heart attack.

Obesity also has the tendency to lead to heart failure. This is a deliberate condition wherein the heart cannot pump enough blood to appropriate the body with the right amount of blood supply.

Type 2 Diabetes. Diabetes is a disease wherein the blood glucose or sugar levels are too high. Typically, our body has the ability to break down the foods we eat into glucose and carries it to our cells. The cells need the help of a hormone called insulin to break down glucose into energy.

In persons with Type two diabetes, the hormone is not fully utilized in breaking down glucose. Initially, the body behaves by making more insulin but over time it cannot produce enough insulin to control blood sugar.

So how can you tell if your weight is more than what you should have?

Gaining a few extra pounds every year does not have an intrinsic effect but the accumulation of it over time does. To tell whether you are overweight, there are two elements to consider. One is your body mass index or the measure of your weight in relation to your height and your waist size in inches.

A normal body mass index has typically been defined as eighteen-point five to twenty-four-point nine percent, or if you are overweight it is twenty-five to twenty-nine point nine percent. If your BMI is more than that, then it's considered obesity already. Your waist size also has to do with the risks of health problems. Women with a waist size of more than thirty-five inches and men with a waist size of more than forty inches tend to gravitate towards developing health and obesity problems.

Case Study: Low Libido Due to Being Overweight

This is a case study of a forty-five-year-old woman with low libido. When a woman's desire to have sexual intercourse or make love with her partner has decreased significantly, she could be experiencing health concerns that may involve her emotional, physical, and mental wellbeing. If not treated immediately, lack of sexual desire could lead to relationship issues and lifestyle problems.

Several factors can be considered in the event of sexual dysfunction in women, that includes job stress, reproductive system problems, diseases, medications, hormonal imbalance, lifestyle, menopausal period, a lack of self-esteem, sexual abuse, and problems with her physical image.

Throughout the whole treatment, we were able to reveal that her sexual dysfunction was a result of her thyroid problem, which eventually led her to become overweight— lack of sexual desire is only a result of her original health concern. However, by undergoing necessary treatments, the patient showed successful recovery.

Weight… It Might Be your Thyroid – Dr. Michael Scott

Patient's symptoms and diagnosis:

This woman had thyroid problems, candida overgrowth, and Gastroesophageal Reflux Disease (GERD) in the past. She complained that she was often sluggish and tired.

For almost a year, she hadn't had any sex nor was she interested in having sexual intercourse. She was working as a corporate executive, which is a stressful job especially for a person of her age. People, women especially, surrounded with huge responsibilities at home and in work tend to have a decline in hormones, increased weight and stress levels, and eventually a loss of interest in sex. They often suffer both mental and physical inconveniences, which can lead to sexual dysfunction.

Add to all these the fact that she was fifteen to twenty pounds overweight.

I had her go through different medical tests to see the underlying reason of her problems. I analyzed her stool and checked her thyroid panels and gut. Genes were also assessed to know if her family had any history of the said disorder. At first, I believed that she was experiencing a much bigger problem than her sexual dysfunction and that this problem was also the reason of her sexual dysfunction—being overweight due to thyroid problems.

Weight… It Might Be your Thyroid – Dr. Michael Scott

And my presumption was right when I saw that the patient's T3 levels were excessively low and her reverse T3 levels were extremely high.

We'll expand more about how T3 or triiodothyronine affects weight loss and weight gain, but to explain briefly about this particular patient's case, T3 is a thyroid hormone that regulates the body's metabolism. When imbalanced, weight gain is one of the possible effects that could immediately occur to the person. It is given that the patient had a high production of reversed T3, which is a consequence of the body not being able to convert T4 to T3. When there is an excess supply of T4, the body will soon convert it to reverse T3. Once the thyroid releases the T4 hormone, it should be converted into an active form.

Normally, your system should be converting the majority of T4 to T3 and a much smaller amount of T4 to reverse T3; however, due to several factors such as job, stress, and lifestyle, these conversions do not happen all the time. More often, there would be a much higher conversion to reverse T3 while T3 remains significantly low, and these conversions lead to several health problems.

The treatment plan:

Seeing that the patient's history of thyroid problems had not been fully treated, I focused on balancing her thyroid hormones. I also recommended her to follow a detox plan which would clean her gut and fix any problems in her stomach. The patient was also given supplements and multivitamins that were high in selenium—a vitamin that can help bring back the normal conversion of T4 to T3.

Alongside with cleaning her gut and fixing her thyroid, I advised her to follow a three-minute a day, three days a week exercise plan, which comprises of interval and resistance training with weights. This workout is intended to build her muscles, heat up core temperature, and speed up her metabolism. Her exercise regime worked her large muscle groups that helped her body to need more energy and thus, burn more calories even after exercise. As this patient was working at a time-constraint schedule and huge responsibilities in the office, the goal was to give her an exercise program that did not consume much of her time but was also effective and focused on her health problem. This patient, by the way, was not doing any exercise programs in the past, so giving her a three-minute a day schedule was the best and most efficient way to treat her medical concerns.

Results / Outcome:

Within three months of gradually following my advice, she lost 12 pounds, her T3 was back in range, and most importantly, she was having sex on a regular basis—which was her first problem when she came into the office. Little did she know, it was only her thyroid that was compromising her libido.

Conclusion:

By implementing simple life changes into our daily routines, we can make the body go back to its natural function. You just have to follow activities the body is inclined to do, not taking advantage and going beyond its limits because when your body's hormones become imbalanced, you will experience several health problems. Whatever your situation is, whether you are bombarded with duties in your home, relationship, or work, do not in any way neglect your health as it is your foundation to work on your responsibilities. Without good health, you can do nothing.

Get a Thyroid Test

A thyroid test is often done to evaluate the function of the thyroid gland. The thyroid is a large ductless gland located at the lower front of the neck that makes thyroid hormones secreted in the blood and carried out to all tissues within the body. The thyroid mainly aids in the regulation of body energy and helps major organs in the body including the heart, muscles and lungs function as normal as they should.

Getting a thyroid test can be beneficial in determining the cause of your weight gain. Hypothyroidism can often be the cause in such cases. A person can experience weight gain, dry skin, constipation, fatigue and other symptoms like menstrual irregularity in women.

Practitioners to evaluate thyroid functions and symptoms of thyroid disorder often do a test known as the thyroid-stimulating hormone test or TSH. TSH is formed by the pituitary gland; a tiny organ that sits below the brain and behind the sinus cavity. It is the body's reaction system in maintaining stable amounts of thyroid hormones such as thyroxine T4 and triiodothyronine (T3) present in the blood to help regulate the body's use of energy.

Weight Loss and Detox

Detoxification is a natural bodily process. It is an automatic response in eliminating and counterbalancing toxins through the colon, kidneys, lungs and other vital organs of our body. Regrettably, our body nowadays has a hard time of trying to get rid of bodily toxins because of the pollution in the air, the chemical contamination of the food and water we take in, and other causes which keeps our bodies having such a hard time maintaining the process.

Our body system was once adept to naturally cleaning out nonessential substances that penetrate our body but are now fully overburdened to the point where toxic materials rest inside our tissues. Our body's natural reaction is to isolate and envelop these dangerous substances with mucous and fat so that they will not cause an imbalance or bring about an immune response.

Detoxification also assists in weight loss, not only does it help you get rid of toxins and free radicals, but helps you cut off those excessively saturated foods which lead to enormous weight gain. A good detox plan involves more fruits and vegetables needed by the body to cleanse itself of harmful toxins and body fat. The detox process also forces you to form good healthy habits, which can have a long-term effect on the body and a drastic reduction in calorie consumption.

Use of Probiotics in Digestion

Using live microorganisms help in digestion and studies have shown that the use of some bacteria has been proven to help with weight loss and belly fat. These friendly bacteria help in breaking down fiber that the body cannot digest turning them into useful short chain fatty acids like butyrate which is beneficial for the colon.

Studies have proven that people with normal weight bear different gut bacteria than overweight and obese people. Body weight, as studies have shown, has a close relation with the balance of two families of microorganisms, namely the bacteroidetes and firmicutes. People with weight problems have more firmicutes and fewer bacteroidetes than people with normal weight. The research also suggests that good bacteria play a crucial role in regulating body weight.

Probiotics and certain bacteria such as those of the Lactobacillus family are also seen as beneficial in fighting obesity because they help release the appetite reducing hormone GLP-1 and aid in burning fats and calories. It also increases the secretion of the protein ANGPTL4 that decreases fat storage within the body. Certain strains from the Lactobacillus family help lose weight and body fats, like Lactobacillus fermentum and Lactobacillus amylovorus which helps reduce body fat when ingested over a period of time. Clinical studies in Japanese adults have shown Lactobacillus gasseri to be effective in promoting weight loss.

Eat right to burn fats

There are certain foods that do not only make your stomach full but also burns fats. These have been seen as the superfoods to lose those excess fats and spare tires. Having a diet that is both rich in vitamins and fiber will remove the temptation of craving and eating sugary and unhealthy foods. It also boosts your metabolism.

A few of the foods you can choose are oatmeal as it stays in the stomach for hours. It allows you to go on with your activity without having to take in much more than you need. Almonds are a better choice than rice cakes, which pack more calories. Getting off saturated oils and choosing avocado or olive oil also helps to maintain your weight. They keep your cholesterol under control and help satisfy your cravings.

Vitamin B12, which helps metabolize fat can be found in eggs. Research has been found to show that people who ate eggs for breakfast lost more weight than those who ate bread. Berries are also packed with a lot of fiber and supplemental sugar.

Beans and legumes are known to be low in calories and high in fiber and protein. They can help you lose weight and shape up. Lean fish and meat also are good sources of protein for losing weight. The body burns more calories digesting proteins than fats or carbohydrates. Salmon and tuna are also rich in Omega-3 which help counter stress. Whole grains are essentially great for the body; they contain more fiber and keep you on the go.

Antioxidant foods such as those rich in betacarotene, vitamin A, C and E, and lycopene are found in most fruits and vegetables. They help reconstruct the cells from toxins and free radicals and can be taken with most supplements available in the market.

Foods and eating habits that are bad for your weight

It's quite easy to spot a food that increases your weight gain. More often than not, it is what we crave. These foods are those rich in calories and pack on tons of fats.

Synthetic foods are a staple item that everyone has. Almost everyone eats processed meat, not only are they readily available, but they have health risks that include bloating your belly and heightening your risk for diabetes. Bacon, hot dogs, sausages, and other deli meat have nitrates that inhibit the body's natural ability to process sugar. It also increases your chances of contracting thyroid and colon cancer. They are also packed with high sodium content that is a known contributor to hypertension that can make you bloat and cause the development of heart ailments.

Diet sodas are also closely linked to obesity as they contain synthetic estrogen that is used to modify the plastic linings of the can, and contain caramel colorants that cause cancers in humans. Some have been studied to contain BVO, a flame-arresting agent often used in rocket fuel. It is seen as the cause for infertility and other thyroid hormonal problems. Mostly all of these beverages contain an artificial sweetener that leads to an elevated sugar level and burdens the liver to create excessive fats.

Having bad eating habits also plays a role for not losing those pounds; an example of this would be trying to finish your food fast. A hectic schedule would often force us to eat faster than we normally would. This is a bad habit, as the food is not fully digested by our digestive system.

Skipping meals is another problem, as it does not save you calories. Instead, you end up consuming more calories in the course of the day to compensate for skipping a meal. Eat your meals on time and aim for three meals a day. Do not skip them; especially breakfast as it is during the daytime where you need the most energy.

Calories from liquid drinks also have to do with your weight gain. Even though you might have control over the foods you eat and the amount you take in, liquid calories from sweetened juices, coffee, cream and sugar, smoothies and alcohol adds up to your intake of calories per day. Instead, you can shift to beverages that are unadulterated like water and vegetable juices.

Using oversized portions like they serve in restaurants and doing the same thing at home also has an impact on weight gain. Instead, you can use smaller plates and bowls at home and regularly use a measuring cup to limit the amount of your food intake.

Thyroid Medications for Weight Loss

The thyroid's function always has an effect on the person's metabolism and weight gain can be a common sign that there is an underlying problem with the thyroid. Hypothyroidism is often associated with weight gain.

Hypothyroidism is a common disorder wherein the thyroid gland does not create enough thyroid hormone. The most frequent cause of the disorder is thyroiditis, or an autoimmune disorder, wherein the body attacks the thyroid gland. This can be caused by a viral infection.

There are also certain causes of this disorder including radiation therapy when treating cancer where radiation is required around the neck area. The therapy damages cells within the thyroid gland that makes it hard to produce hormones. Radioactive iodine treatment is also seen as one cause of this disorder. This is a treatment that most people with an overactive thyroid undergo. It destroys cells in the thyroid gland.

Having a high or low BMR, or Basal Metabolic Rate, a way to measure the amount of oxygen used by the body over an appropriate amount of time, is often linked to the adjustment in energy balance.

Other hormones, neurotransmitters and proteins are also involved in the distribution of body fat and its storage. This includes insulin, leptin, neuropeptide Y, and inflammatory proteins like interleukin 6.

Leptin is a hormone formed in the fat cells of the body that helps regulate and maintain body weight. It also has an effect on the thyroid. Leptin is responsible for control of your organ's fat balance and whether you need to eat more or stop at a low-metabolism endurance state. Having a high leptin level means having more fat cells. As your metabolism becomes gradually slower, your Thyroid Stimulating Hormone or TSH increases and dictates to your thyroid to create more thyroid hormones.

Serotonin also plays a major role with hypothyroidism. Serotonin is a neurotransmitter that instructs you to stop eating. When the body does not secrete a certain amount of serotonin, it leads to certain conditions such as depression and lessens that signal that tells you to stop eating. Thus, a food craving is aggravated and can build up to weight gain and hypothyroidism.

The Role of Exercise on Weight Loss

Physical activity and exercise are two different things. Physical activities are movements that are carried out and require energy, while, exercise is structured, repetitive and premeditated movements to maintain physical health.

Studies have sufficiently proven that exercise has helped in contributing to overall well-being and health. It has a significant role in influencing energy metabolism in individuals and helps circulate thyroid hormones in the body.

For people who are suffering hypothyroidism, experts advise to take low-impact aerobic exercise training. These forms of exercises elevate your heart rate without putting too much pressure on your joints. A daily regimen of exercises accelerates your heart rate, which is beneficial to the body. It increases the circulation of hormones such as thyroxine, triiodothyronine and other thyroid stimulating hormones. It also helps combat stress related problems.

Exercises such as lunges, push-ups and leg raises can be beneficial for people who have hypothyroidism as they counter the possibility of gaining excessive weight. A daily regimen of exercise builds muscle mass, burns calories and strengthens your muscle.

The best exercises for thyroid problems are squats, where you stand straight up and bend your knees until you are in a sitting position. You can also do one-leg deadlifts. Hold onto something for balance while keeping one hand laid back in front of your thigh. Then push your hips as far as you can, until your hand comes in contact with the ground. Then you can come back up. This is just one of several exercises you can do to help build a stronger and healthier metabolism.

Sleep and Weight Loss

There are several benefits of getting good rest. It does not only invigorate the body, but helps to repair damaged cells. Sleep deprivation ultimately leads to different complications that involve not only the mental well-being the physical aspect as well.

Weight… It Might Be your Thyroid – Dr. Michael Scott

Studies have shown that sleep deprivation leads to obesity and statistics have shown that they are closely related. A study using volunteers who were given different sleeping patterns but the same diet regimen, revealed that those who were given an ample amount of rest had a decrease in body fat that was nearly cut in half due to sleep. Meanwhile, those who did not get adequate sleep had their fat loss cut in half. Additionally, those who were deprived felt incomparably hungrier, were less gratified after meals, and didn't have the energy to exercise.

Inadequate sleep also changes your fat cells when the body is in need of a good rest. It experiences a process that is termed metabolic grogginess. Metabolic grogginess happens when the hormones that control your fat cells do not behave the way they should. This happens when your body's capacity to use insulin shifts into uncontrollable disruption.

The problem with metabolic grogginess is the effectiveness of insulin functioning well. When it does not function as intended, fat cells expel fatty acids into the blood stream and prohibit the use of insulin. If you become more insulin resistant, lipids distribute in the blood streams causing the body to make more sugar. Ultimately, that extra sugar ends up storing in fat cells in the awry places like the liver. This is how you are inclined to get fat and diseases like diabetes.

Another is the secretion of hormones such as leptin and ghrelin. Leptin is the hormone we spoke about earlier that is formed in the fat cells. The less leptin your body makes, the hungrier you feel. The more ghrelin your body makes, the more you prompt hunger while also decreasing the amount of your metabolism, which again increases your storage of fat.

By way of explanation, you need to take control of your body's leptin and ghrelin production in order to lose weight although, sleep deprivation makes that virtually impossible. Published studies have shown that not getting enough sleep stimulates an area in your brain that increases the need for food while also suppressing leptin and invigorating the overproduction of the hormone ghrelin.

Researchers have also discovered how sleep deprivation scts up an internal battle that makes weight loss practically impossible. When a person does not get good enough sleep, the cortisol level rises. Cortisol is a stress hormone that is often associated with fat gain. Cortisol also activates a part of your brain that makes you crave for food. At the same time, sleep deprivation forces your body to create more ghrelin. The combination of both ghrelin and high levels of cortisol closes down areas in your brain that leave you satisfied after a meal. What's more alarming is that it also pushes you to the path of craving foods you shouldn't eat.

Weight... It Might Be your Thyroid – Dr. Michael Scott

In a separate finding, it was also established that not getting enough sleep impairs activity in your frontal lobe, the body part that manages complex decision making.

THE BIG LIE

The Metabolism Slows Down at a Certain Age

Most of us believe that as people age, metabolism automatically slows down which results in weight gain. In fact, statistics show that adults have been particularly hard hit by the so-called worldwide epidemic of obesity.

According to a 2009-2010 study published in the Journal of American Medical Association, the United States alone saw a thirty-five-percent increase in obesity in adults and another sixty-seven-percent increase for those who are considered bordering between overweight and obesity. What is even more alarming is that the numbers of those obese and overweight continues to rise as the distribution of body mass index (BMI) has changed.

The National Health and Nutrition Examination Survey conducted a follow-up survey among adults whose ages were between twenty-five and forty-four-years old. In the newer polls, the health authority found that men gained about three-point-four percent of their body weight every ten years while women got heavier with five-point-two percent added to their weight for the same duration.

Weight… It Might Be your Thyroid – Dr. Michael Scott

Practicing pediatrician, registered dietitian, and ACE Fit senior consultant Dr. Natalie Digate Muth said metabolism and age both may have played significant roles that resulted in these alarming numbers. As we age, people have a tendency to become less active which, in turn, results in a decrease in the calories we burn.

Citing a study that evaluated the total energy expenditure (TEE) which is equal to the sum of the amount of calories burned through metabolism, physical activity, and the energy needed to digest and absorb food, Dr. Muth confirmed that energy expenditure decreases as a person grows older.

We've heard this many times before but put in a different way. I've had patients come to me after being told, "You've reached 40 years old. Your metabolism automatically slows down now".

I agree with Dr. Muth, to an extent. Saying that a person's metabolism slows because he is forty years old implies that a person's age is the main reason why his metabolism functions slower than it should.

"If that were true, everyone over forty should be overweight. The fact is that metabolism can slow down regardless of a person's age,".

The key to understanding why most adults, at a particular age, have slowed metabolism is to decipher what the process of metabolism is all about and what factors contribute to its diminishing performance.

What is Metabolism?

Metabolism is the bodily process that not only explains how the body burns up the calories we eat but also tackles how the body converts these foods into proteins at a cellular level. This is called protein synthesis and is controlled by the endocrine system.

The endocrine system is mainly composed of the glands that control the body's hormone production. The thyroid gland is among these and is known to be the ruler of the body's metabolic process because it produces hormones called the tri-iodothyronine or T3, and the thyroxine or T4.

According to Endocrine Web, the thyroid works as the metabolism regulator by extracting iodine from the blood and incorporating it into the thyroid to make its hormones. Because of this, the decrease of production of such hormones causes slowed metabolism.

Weight Gain, Metabolism and the Thyroid Glands

Weight gain is usually caused by slowed metabolism that resulted from bad eating habits. As we age, we start to develop or have already developed specific eating habits that are not conducive to maintaining the weight we want.

But aside from that, one reason why we gain so much weight over the years is because our bodies are exposed to toxins that prevent the endocrine system from working at its maximum. Such toxins can come from our environment as well as the things we consume (eat and drink).

But don't fret, once metabolism is slowed in a regular adult, it can still be improved by ten percent to thirty percent. It is just a matter of regulating how the body converts thyroid hormone by making sure that the body's conversion network is working at its maximum capability. One of the process with which this can be achieved is called detox.

Increasing Metabolism through Detox

A regular adult has at least one of seven hundred types of toxins in his body depending on where he lives. It can be from pollution, toothpaste, dry cleaning or specific kinds of fabrics. Unless you live in a bubble, you are exposed to toxins.

This is why every single person, no matter how strict they are in their diet and lifestyle should undergo detoxification to remove these toxins and other impurities from their body. It is the function of the liver to package these toxins and remove them from our body. However, there are instances when the liver can no longer process the amount of toxins the body absorbs.

This is where the detoxification process comes in. Basically, detoxification entails eating the right food and getting rid of what you already ate.

How to Detoxify

According to Gaiam Life, a good detoxification process should include:

- fasting to allow the organs to rest

- stimulating the liver to drive the toxins out of the body

- promoting digestion and elimination of toxins through the liver, intestines, kidneys and skin

- improve blood circulation

- refuel the body with healthy foods that are rich in nutrients

The first step in detoxifying is lightening up your load. This simply means removing any possible source of toxins such as alcohol, coffee and cigarettes, as well as foods that are high in saturated fats and sources of refined sugars.

Aside from that, it is also important that the person undergoing detox minimize contact with chemical-based compounds like household cleaners and personal health care products. This includes shampoos, bath soaps, cleansers, deodorants, and even your toothpaste. Try substituting these synthetic products with brands that are labeled "All-Natural" or "a hundred percent Natural".

Quick Tip: In between detox, you should drink plenty of water to flush your cells. It is best that you avoid sodas and juices.

Case Study: Living a Healthy Lifestyle but Having a Hard Time Losing Weight

This next case study is about a sixty-one-year old woman who is doing perfectly well with her health but she could not lose any of her extra weight. There have been claims that people who are in their forties and onward are struggling at losing weight especially if they have gone past their menopausal period. Several factors can be considered as to why losing weight gets harder as we age and these include aging muscles, hormonal changes, inability to flex muscles, lifestyle changes, diseases, injury, and bodily changes.

As our body gets older, our muscle tissues shrink; wear and tear. And when the muscle starts to diminish, burning calories gets much more difficult, and unburned calories eventually become unwanted fat and extra pounds.

The problem with reaching the menopausal stage is that it changes where fat is usually stored. With this, people in their fifties start to accumulate more fat in their hips, thighs, stomach, and arms. During this stage, a person will also decrease one's daily activities and slow down metabolism. Even doing exercises such as walking, swimming, lifting, and running will become a problem. Thus, low-impact tasks are not enough to help a person build muscle, burn calories, and lose weight. Breathing, fatigue, and joint problems are also contributing factors why seniors do not want to move too much in their sixties.

Bodily changes and diseases are also a big culprit why weight loss is such a struggle during our golden years. I found out that, with this particular senior woman and her weight loss problem, the culprit wasn't just her age it was her thyroid. Through simple lifestyle tweaks, the lady gradually regained her youthful energy and eventually lost her extra weight.

Patient's signs and symptoms

This sixty-one-year-old woman is married to a physician and has also worked for a physician. She said she was following a holistic lifestyle. She was eating right and doing regular and intense exercise, particularly, racquetball. She thought she was doing perfect because of her healthy lifestyle, but wondered why she could not lose any weight at all despite her extreme exercise regime. She came into my clinic with her husband, who is also her longtime racquetball opponent. Immediately, when she told me of her problems and her lifestyle, I suspected that it was her thyroid that was causing her to struggle with losing weight. Though her physician husband didn't believe this claim I guaranteed him that my suspicions were true.

As suggested we checked her thyroid panels and found that she had very low T3 which was only point eight and a high reverse T3 level of twenty-four. Her TT4 was also elevated. The doctor saw that the patient was having conversion problems with T4 to T3. She was thirty-four pounds overweight and also suffering from plantar fasciitis. The patient said that seven days before she visited my office she and her husband had already slowed down the amount of time they played racquetball due to her heel pain.

The treatment plan

I had the patient follow a medical liver detox. She was also given a multivitamin high in selenium, medium chain triglyceride coconut oil and protein shakes to speed metabolism, and resistant starch, which improves insulin sensitivity. She also cut out carbs and refined sugar in her diet. Lastly, she had to follow a regular exercise routine at the gym three minutes a day, three days a week. However, her choice of exercise was to play racquetball and that was fine as long as she was doing any form of exercise.

My first goal was to clean her gut and normalize the release of thyroid hormones in her body by removing excess wastes that had been stored in her liver, kidneys, and colon for years. The second goal was to speed up her metabolism, and third was to help her lose weight.

Results / Outcome

After two months of regularly following her treatment plan the patient's thyroid hormone conversion had been normalized and her plantar fasciitis had almost completely subsided. She also noticed that she felt lighter and happier. And most importantly, she lost weight. After two months of eating right, exercising, and detoxing, she had already lost nine pounds. A few months later, she lost twenty-four pounds more.

Conclusion

No matter what your age, you can still lose weight provided that you're doing it right. You need to find out first the underlying reason for your weight gain and then follow a weight loss program that will work for you.

The Speed of Metabolism

People often complain about getting fat and blame their slowed metabolism for it. This is true in a sense, but what about those people who do not ever gain weight no matter what they eat?

The fact is, even those who are lucky enough to still have their metabolism working at its peak despite their bad eating habits are still not safe from getting fat.

This is because no matter how admirable their metabolism is, it does not guarantee them from having weight gain problems if they continue with their bad eating habits. The best way is still to eat the right food, do right by our liver and there should be no weight gain problem at all.

Slowed metabolism has adverse effects on the body not only with respect to our appearance but also our overall health. Our bodies are programmed to hold on to fat. Exercising alone won't get your metabolism up and running. Even if you jog until your tongue is hanging, your body will still retain fats that will serve as your energy reserves because it is programmed to do so. The thing you should focus on is your favorite sweetener: sugar.

Why Sugar is Bad for Weight Loss

Sugar is the generalized term used for the sweet, short-chain, soluble carbohydrates that are added to our food for better taste. According to Food.com, it was once called "white gold" and considered a luxury that was available only for the wealthy and traded in blocks not in granule form. Now, sugar comes in different textures, colors, consistencies and flavor.

In nutrition and medicine, however, "sugar" refers to the substance produced from breaking down the food that we eat—this is the so-called glucose.

Glucose is a simple sugar that is generally referred to as humans' and other animals' energy source. Carbohydrates and saccharides are converted into sugar from the foods we eat and turned into energy. However, it has become more popular nowadays for its association with the chronic disease diabetes.

Foods That Contain Sugar or Glucose

There are quite a number of foods that have high sugar content, many of which may still be in your diet. In fact, WebMD revealed foods that have shockingly high levels of sugar in them.

"Just because there's a nutrition-oriented statement on the package (like 'contains whole grain,' 'excellent source of calcium,' 'fat-free,' 'a hundred percent juice' or 'twenty-five percent less sugar') doesn't mean it doesn't contain a shocking amount of sugar," the health site explained.

Shockingly, the list of sugary foods included things that many people believed to be a healthier substitute for regular food such as canned or packaged fruits, diet cereal bars, breakfast cereals, instant hot cereals and yogurt. It has some widely favored snacks like muffins, and cakes as well as sauces for spaghetti and barbecue.

The beverages included in the list included plain and flavored milk drinks, juices (both natural and processed), instant tea or bottled tea, vitamin and energy drinks, and instant cocoa. Processed and frozen viands also crowded the list.

In the United States, there are a lot of processed foods and beverages that are labeled with "No Sugar" but actually have other ingredients that can be broken down into glucose such as corn syrup. This kind of sweetener has high-fructose content that is still broken down into glucose once processed by the body.

Don't get the wrong idea. It is not really bad to have carbohydrates in your diet as long as it is within the advisable limits. Unfortunately, many people have a tendency to eat foods such as pasta with others that also contain high levels of carbohydrate such as bread, leaving their meals unbalanced. Even worse, they eat dessert, which, again, contains a lot of sugar after that high-glucose meal.

Case Study: Seemingly Healthy Foods That Are Doing More Harm Than Good

This next case study is about a thirty-nine-year-old woman who thought she was eating right. However, she noticed that she was not losing weight, rather, she was gaining weight despite her healthy food choices. Diet coke, zero percent trans-fat, no added sugar, no MSG, processed low-fat, "fruit" juices, "whole" wheat, sports drink, low-carb junk food, processed "organic" food, gluten-free junk food, "whole grain" breakfast cereal—everyone has been fooled by these crazy, manipulative, and deceitful advertisements. And these are what this next client had been dealing with together with her entire family.

Truth is, ninety percent of food brands that you see in the grocery stands are laden with chemicals that are not in any way good for you. All of the phrases that were mentioned above, which we often see in food labels, are false advertisements you don't want to fall into. When we read a healthy word on a food label, we immediately assume that it is, in the real sense, healthy. However, this is not always the case. Say for example, granola.

Back in the sixty when GMO foods and food chemicals were not so rampant, we could, in fact, claim that granola was a healthier food choice compared to candies and heavily sugared breakfast cereals. But with today's food standards, you don't even know what your granola is made of. All of the ingredients that you don't recognize are just sheer sugar, salt, and fat. In this case, a granola, in today's time, is just as bad as candy and junk food.

This food may contain a tiny amount of vitamins and minerals, but with the amount of sugar and salt contained in it, the bad stuff seems to outweigh the good stuff.

This next patient thought she was eating right and was providing healthy food to her family. But with a little guidance, she learned how to make better food choices.

The patient

A forty five years old woman and a mother of three children was having a hard time losing weight despite the "healthy" food she provided on the table. She asked for help figuring out why she was not losing any weight. Being a good friend mine I decided to visit her house to see what was happening, and immediately upon checking her kitchen cabinets, I found the problem.

Her pantry and refrigerator were loaded with snacks and foods that had the food labels mentioned earlier. She had boxes of cereals, bags of "healthy" chips, peanut butter that had twelve ingredients, jelly, cured bacon, Ramen noodles, cookies, and fruit snacks—every food that proclaims to be healthy. She was the one who did the grocery shopping and she decided what went into her family's body—all because she thought she knew how to choose better food options. What she did not know was that what they were eating was all processed food that had been loaded with chemicals, sugar, salt, hydrogenated oil, and bad saturated fat.

Her kids ages thirteen, eleven, and nine, are all into sports at their schools and these junk foods were what they had been consuming for years. Their coach, as the mother told me, said that she should make sure her kids were eating more carbs as they are into so many physical activities. While this may be true, the problem lies in the choice of carbs the patient was making for her family.

This patient, by the way, had also been diagnosed with diabetes before. She was thirty-four pounds overweight. Her feet and skin were dry and her body was bloated—warning signs that she had been dehydrated by the amount of salt and sugar from the processed foods she had been eating.

The treatment plan

Truth is, I just educated the family how to differentiate healthy food from unhealthy food. She and I sat down with her family and discussed how to pick the right peanut butter from a peanut butter with ingredients they'd never heard of; how to choose real fruit from fruit snacks bought in the grocery stands; how to understand food labels; and how to portion size their meals. The family was also encouraged to eat home-cooked meals instead of buying fast food.

Her thyroid was not checked because the problem was only about the family's food choices. She just had to change her diet, make healthier food choices, and follow a healthier lifestyle wherein the family should embrace home-cooked meals and snacks more often.

Results / Outcomes

Within two months, just by changing her food choices, she lost twenty-five pounds. Alongside switching to a healthier lifestyle, she started doing marathons. Her insulin was also back in the normal range which prevented sugar from becoming fat and helped her regulate her diabetes.

Conclusion

Following a healthy lifestyle is not all about eating what the food label says is healthy. It's all about going back to what's natural and healthy for your body. It's about preparing a healthier menu. It's about planning, about portion sizing, about control. It's about getting your body back to its natural function.

If you want to drink fruit juice, find time to prepare your own beverage. Don't be fooled by a "100%" orange juice claim on the label. You know it's not all true. And when you drink your own prepared fruit juice, pay attention to your serving size. The fruit itself also has sugar in it, and while it's a much better option than refined sugar, too much of this type of sugar can also be unhealthy.

Control the demands of your tongue and stomach and educate your senses to choose a healthier alternative. This practice will clean your stomach from the toxins you have been consuming in the past. When you see a potato snack on the shelf, tell your mind and tongue that a real potato is a much better option. Now tell your eyes to look for a real potato. Help yourself and be in command of your senses. If you do this on a regular basis, it will be automatic to your mind and senses to choose healthier foods without you commanding them. It becomes natural.

Be mindful of your activities and what you put in your mouth. Put love in everything that you do so you won't be lazy doing things that may need your time such as cooking, educating yourself, and switching to a holistic lifestyle. If you need help, call for professional help. If you are surrounded with your family, get them involved and tell them your goals so they can help you achieve them.

Make a conscious plan and conscious decision to work on your plan. This is a life-changing event and it needs you to be present in the moment.

Fruits and Kids

Another popular belief that people should reconsider is the effects of putting too much fruit in their body. Parents often give their children fruits because of the common notion that fruits, like vegetables, are best snacks for their children.

While it is filled with vitamins, including too many fruits in your child's diet may have negative effects for his metabolism because these scrumptious snacks are also found to have high sugar content. Because of this, eating more fruits or drinking their juices—even ones squeezed directly from them—requires more work from liver.

While kids can process sugars better than adults, because their organs are still operating at their peak, giving them more high-sugar foods and drinks than they should at an early age can cause too much stress on their pancreases. Because it has to function at a high level all the time, children who eat too much fruit end up with insulin resistance or Type 2 Diabetes.

Consuming the Right Kind of Calories

After understanding which foods are good for you and which are not, it is also important that you learn how to discern the right king of calorie for your body. Adhering to the advised daily calorie intake may still cause a person to gain unwanted weight. To explain further, here is an example of how two people could experience different effects if they eat two different diet combinations even with the same amount of calories.

Sample:

Person A – moderate protein, high fat, very low or no carbs

Person B – moderate to high carb, low fat, moderate protein

Both women, who are under two-thousand-calorie diets for thirty days, will show different results. However, one of them will gain weight, while the other will lose weight.

After thirty days, Person A will lose weight while Person B will gain weight. This is because the body uses certain calories for energy and other biological functions. While the body requires sugar for energy, it still needs other nutrients to accomplish all biological processes each day.

When the body has low sugar, it automatically adapts and finds another energy source to keep you up and running.

This is when the liver produces a substance called "ketones." These are the acids produced as your back up energy source when sugar supply in the blood is too low.

Because Person A has high levels of fat intake in his diet, his body can produce enough ketones to supplement the lack of sugar from his low carb diet. Meanwhile, Person B who has a high carb diet uses up only a portion of the sugar from the food he ate but retains some that later accumulates inside her fat cells and makes her look fat.

Consuming a lot of sugar means you will have excess weight. Once sugar is decreased or removed from the diet, the body then proceeds to use up the remaining sugar that is stored in the body for energy. After that, if a person proceeds to a high fat diet but keeps low or no sugar, his body adapts and uses up the excess fat.

The bottom line is: once you put sugar in the body, it uses it up for energy and leaves the fat to accumulate but if the body detects no sugar, it converts fat into energy and burns it up.

It is important to supplement your sugar intake so as to prevent your body from needing to produce too many ketones for your energy source. This is because too many ketones may imply that you have some serious underlying medical conditions such as ketoacidosis in which case you should seek the help of a medical professional.

Health-line defines ketones as "the acids made when your body begins using fat instead of carbohydrates for energy." According to the site, this substance is produced when the body does not have enough insulin supply to pump up sugar to the blood for distribution to the different organs of your body. Its presence in the body is also described to be normal provided that you don't already have diabetes.

You should test your ketone level if:

- your blood glucose level goes over three-hundred

- your skin is either flushed or pale

- you experience symptoms such as nausea, vomiting, or abdominal pain without being sick with other illnesses

- you have illness, injuries, or infections which can cause sudden high blood glucose

- you have very little energy and/or feel confused

- you have dry mouth or feel thirstier than usual

- you have difficulty breathing

- your breath smells "fruity"

Gaining "Fat"

It is important to understand that looking "fat" does not necessarily result from eating fatty foods. In fact, often times people who look rounder than others usually appear that way because of their high-sugar diet. Because they store more carbohydrates than they can use up, the fat in their bodies-their energy reserves-remain unused.

Even if you don't look closely, you'll surely notice that certain parts of our bodies "inflate" faster than the others. If you notice, our abdomen, thighs, and the back of our necks tend to become fatter, quicker. This is because those parts have more fat cells in them.

Fat cells are the cells that become the storage facility for excess sugar that is not used up by the body. When filled with sugar, the fat cells expand like balloons. The more sugar absorbed in them, the bigger they get. This is the reason why we look "fat."

This also debunks the common misconception that fat in our food per se is the one causing all the bad. In fact, I'd like to emphasize that fat is actually good for the body. It is the sugar that you might want to control. When sugar is gradually used up when a person goes on a low carb diet, the fat cells then deflate, thereby making the person become leaner.

Maintaining Your Weight

To lessen the glucose in the body, it is important to look into diet options that contain low carb and high fat foods. Talking simply, listed below are foods that are "safe" for your low carb diet and those which aren't:

Eat: Meat, fish, eggs, vegetables growing above ground and natural fats (like butter).

Don't Eat: Sugar, HFCS, starchy foods, wheat, seed oils, trans-fats, 'diet' and low-fat products, and processed foods.

When maintaining a diet regimen, it is important to remember to always read the ingredients list and not rely on the labels. According to the site, some brands labeled as "health foods" are not actually perfect for your low carb diet.

After removing excess sugar that has been stored from your body and burning through the stored and unused fats, you can return to incorporating foods that produce glucose back into your diet. However, if you want to maintain your current weight, you should do so with moderation.

You don't have to splurge because at this point in life, having excess sugar for you to burn, fill your fat cells as well as your muscles, the results could turn for the worst such as diseases like diabetes and many others.

Recommendations

At their early age, parents should teach children to learn to get used to food that is healthier and has lower sugar content. If every parent did this, there will come a time that you see children craving vegetables instead of candies and chocolates.

Meanwhile, adults can start substituting high-carb foods with complex carbs. According to Nutrition MD, complex carbs are dietary starches made of sugar molecules that are "strung together like a necklace or branched like a coil." Foods rich in complex carbs usually contain high fiber.

Here are some examples of complex carbs:

- Green vegetables

- Whole grains and foods made from them, such as oatmeal, pasta, and whole-grain breads

- Starchy vegetables such as potatoes, sweet potatoes, corn, and pumpkin

- Beans, lentils, and peas

The best part about doing this is that you get to absorb the energy you need for your bodily processes with other vitamins and minerals. Plus, you get to lose weight provided you always keep your diet in check.

Points to Remember:

- Regardless of age, it is important to maintain a healthy diet.

- Metabolism can be enhanced through detoxification.

- Age does not necessarily affect metabolism. It is more the person's eating habits.

- Choose the right kind of calories.

- Being "fat" does not mean you should not eat fatty foods. It means you should lessen your carbohydrate intake.

- Choose healthy by examining the food's ingredients and not the label alone.

- Eat complex carbohydrates.

The Thyroid

Weight gain is just a symptom. Once we fix the cause, we fix the symptom. It's simply a matter of finding out what the problem is and fixing it.

Weight gain is a problem that ripples, leaving many other predicaments in its wake. Aside from the well-known physical issues it may cause, it can also ignite psychological ailments in the individual.

This is because people who are considered obese, overweight, or are nearing these conditions become sedentary, which sometimes turn to self-blame and, in worst cases, develops into depression.

Surprisingly, more and more people tend to neglect the importance of monitoring their weight so much so that the issue is now considered to be a bigger problem than world hunger, according to a study published in the British medical journal, The Lancet.

"Obesity and especially severe and morbid obesity, affect many organs and physiological processes. We can deal with some of these, like higher cholesterol or blood pressure, through medicines. But for many others, including diabetes, we don't have effective treatment," the study's lead author Majid Ezzati explained.

Moreover, a lot of people are unaware that most of the time weight gain is a result of issues with a small gland located in a person's throat known as the "thyroid." In this chapter, we will discuss everything you need to know about the thyroid gland and how it affects a person's weight through metabolism.

What is the Thyroid?

The thyroid is part of the endocrine system, located in front of the neck just above the Adam's apple. The thyroid gland is a butterfly-shaped organ that's about two inches long, almost the size of a half-dollar.

According to Endocrine Web, it produces hormones that regulate several functions in the body, including vital ones like breathing, heart rate, muscle strength, menstrual cycles, body temperature, cholesterol levels, and the functions of the peripheral and central nervous systems.

It also regulates the metabolism of every cell in the human body, making it a major player in controlling your body weight.

Thyroid Diseases

Despite its role in the vital processes of the body, the thyroid gland is usually neglected, which typically leads to diseases such as goiter, thyroiditis, hyperthyroidism, hypothyroidism, Grave's disease, cancer, thyroid nodule, thyroid storm, and several others.

Among these ailments, hypothyroidism is the most common reason for weight gain. In fact, weight gain is one of the major signs that a person has hypothyroidism. This condition is characterized by the thyroid's failure to produce enough hormones, which results in an imbalance in chemical reactions in the body.

Some of the most common reasons why the thyroid breaks down are environmental toxins. Toxins, as explained in the previous chapter, can come from the food we eat as well as our surroundings.

There could also be a possible problem with the body's immune system that leads to the anti-bodies attacking the thyroid. This condition is called Hashimoto's thyroiditis, an autoimmune condition where anti-bodies, or the body's defense mechanism, strike the thyroid gland and destroy it.

Another pertinent cause of thyroid diseases is the imbalance in a person's intestinal ecology. According to Smart Publications, your gut houses more than a hundred trillion live bacteria and other microorganisms—often called the "intestinal flora."

These live bacteria are divided into two kinds: the good and the bad. When a person's intestinal flora is predominated by the beneficial bacteria, it is considered healthy. This is because the good bacteria help in some of the vital bodily processes particularly in digestion by producing nutrients such as the Vitamins B2, B5, and B12, and organic acids like lactic acid.

However, when the intestinal ecology is tilted in favor of the bad bacteria, a person's health begins to turn for the worse.

The Hormones and How They Work

The human metabolism process can be compared to a communication process since it involves two glands that are covered by the endocrine system. The thyroid produces hormones that communicate with the cells by traveling through the blood stream after being told to do so by a different hormone produced in the pituitary gland.

Weight… It Might Be your Thyroid – Dr. Michael Scott

The pituitary gland is a pea-sized organ attached to the brain, which is known to control a person's growth and development. It can also be considered the control center for several endocrine glands, including the thyroid.

Here is a simplified step-by-step description on how the process proceeds.

- To make sure that the cells metabolize properly, the pituitary gland produces thyroid stimulating hormone (TSH), which activates the thyroid's hormone-production function.

- From there, the thyroid produces a hormone called thyroxine, also known as T4. The T4 is an inactive hormone that travels through the blood to the cells.

- Upon reaching various organs of the body through the blood stream, the T4 is then converted into the triiodothyronine (T3)

- T3 is the active thyroid hormone that travels through the blood system to the cells to stimulate them to function properly.

The thyroid produces about nighty-seven percent T4 and just three percent T3. However, only a small amount of T3 produced by the thyroid remains in the gland to make sure it functions properly while the rest of it travels with the T4 through the body after the inactive hormone has been converted.

Here is another way of understanding the process as described by Endocrine Web:

"Thyroid hormones are like heat. When the heat gets back to the thermostat, it turns the thermostat off. As the room cools (the thyroid hormone levels drop), the thermostat turns back on (TSH increases) and the furnace produces more heat (thyroid hormones)."

The bottom line is that if any of these hormones are in shortage, the cells will not operate as fast as they need to.

Iodine and the Thyroid Hormones

Iodine is a wondrous mineral that is usually found in salt as well as foods from the sea. It is typically known as the orange tincture used to disinfect scrapes and wounds. However, iodine has another more important role—to help the thyroid to produce the T3 and T4 hormones.

Because the body cannot produce its own supply of iodine, the thyroid's only source of this element is limited to the food we consume. This is why it is imperative that one's diet should have enough iodine content to supply the thyroid.

Aside from salt and seafood, iodine can also be found in dairy products, meat, eggs, as well as certain kinds of bread. People who live in areas that have limited access to the ocean are often exposed to iodine deficiency, which is why experts advise them to take multivitamins with iodine.

Iodine deficiency is something that should not be taken lightly because all its symptoms are directly related to most of the thyroid diseases stated above.

The cells in the thyroid gland are the only ones that can absorb iodine. By combining it with the amino acid known as tyrosine, the thyroid gland converts iodine into the hormones T3 and T4, which are essential for the body's metabolism or the conversion of calories and oxygen to energy.

Thyroid Function Tests

Available tests cover the TSH, T4, T3, Thyroid Peroxidase Antibodies (TPO), Thyroglobulin Antibodies (TGB) and T3 Resin Uptake (T3RU). However, it is imperative that you ask a specialist to interpret them because they are complicated and rely on various conditions that can change the implications of results per individual.

Typically, the first test recommended for patients with weight gain problems to check thyroid function is to measure the level of TSH in the blood. People with an underactive thyroid typically have high levels of TSH because the thyroid is not making enough T3 and/or T4 even if the pituitary gland orders it to produce more. If this is the case, more tests should be conducted. These people usually experience weight gain, lack of energy, and depression. A TSH reading of above two milli-international units of hormone per liter of blood (mIU/L) is worrying because it can be a sign of hypothyroidism.

Meanwhile, people with overactive thyroid, or those with hyperthyroidism, have low levels of TSH because the thyroid is making too much T3 and T4 hormones. They may also experience weight loss, feel high levels of anxiety, tremors, and a sense of being on a high.

Normal TSH test results range between point four and four mIU/L.

The next hormone to be tested after TSH is the T4 with a laboratory process known as the thyroxine test. If the test showed high T4, it is a sign that the patient has overactive thyroid or hyperthyroidism.

After that, the level of the hormone triiodothyronine or T3 is tested, usually after T4 and TSH results that indicate possible hyperthyroidism.

Results above the normal T3 level range of a hundred to two-hundred nanograms of hormone per deciliter of blood implies that a person may have an autoimmune disorder known as Grave's disease. When this happens, the doctor may require the patient to undergo the T3RU or the T3 Resin Uptake test. It determines the level of a hormone known as thyroxin-binding globulin (TBG) which is usually low when T3 is elevated. Do not confuse this with TGB which is a protein produced by the thyroid gland to make T3 and T4 hormones.

If TBG level is high, the patient may have issues with his kidneys or the body may not be getting an ample supply of protein. Meanwhile, if TBG level is high, there is a big chance that the patient also has a high level of estrogen. This may occur during pregnancy, if the patient eats estrogen-rich foods or he is undergoing hormone replacement therapy. It is also an indicator of obesity.

Thyroid and Your Weight

Patients often complain about not being able to lose weight even if they only eat healthy foods and exercise regularly. Oftentimes, weight gain under these circumstances may be due to an issue with the thyroid gland or the hormones it produces.

If the thyroid is not functioning properly, it cannot produce T4 to be converted into T3, which means cells are not being stimulated. Thus, the metabolism is not revved up.

However, there are some instances when the thyroid gland is perfectly fine. In these cases, a medical practitioner will be looking into possible issues with the level of hormones produced by the endocrine system.

Most patients present test results that only measure the levels of TSH and T4 from the thyroid. T4 and TSH work together to stay in equilibrium. The production of TSH is the pituitary gland's way of telling the thyroid to produce more T4. If there is enough T4, the thyroid signals the pituitary gland to stop or reduce the production of TSH. But because the ranges for what is considered normal for both TSH and T4 hormone count are both wide, most test results are within normalcy.

If both TSH and T4 are normal, the problem may be in the T4's conversion to T3. After finding the T4 and TSH results within normal range, most professionals deem the thyroid gland to be fine look for reasons not related to the gland as to why the patient continues to gain weight.

This is where most of the mistake occurs. The problem is that people do not often check the total T3 values among other things to determine if the thyroid is really fine and look elsewhere for answers.

In most cases, the thyroid remains central to the issue because it is the gland that regulates the body's metabolic process. Keep in mind that knowing this should not be the cause of worry since it can be fixed with a simple change in diet or supplementation of thyroid hormones.

After finding out that the conversion from T4 to T3 really is the problem, more tests should be conducted to find out where in the body the conversion process failed. Since most of the conversion is done in the liver, detox may be needed to flush out toxins from the organ.

Additional exams may also be required to check laboratory markers for inflammation. Chronic inflammation in the body can prevent the liver or any other part of the body from producing an enzyme known as deiodinase that converts T4 to T3. It causes problems with cell membranes which makes them fail to function the way they are supposed to.

Natural Endocrine Solutions listed a couple of reasons why the body fails to produce deiodinase.

- Mineral Deficiencies. The activation of enzymes requires minerals such as selenium and zinc. People with low levels of selenium and/or zinc may experience problems with their T4 to T3 conversion.

- Gastrointestinal Issues. Issues with your gut may result in problems with the absorption of the above mentioned minerals necessary for the conversion of T3 to T4. Most of the time, the issue with your gut is a result of predominance of bad bacteria in the body. Having a healthy gut is also important in the conversion process by releasing an enzyme that is responsible for the activation of the T3: the intestinal sulfatase.

- Liver Problems. Since a huge chunk of the body's T4 to T3 conversion occurs in the liver, there is a big chance that problems with the organ can cause disruption or irregularity in the process. Furthermore, the site explained that liver enzyme measurement tests can only rule out the serious issues which do not necessarily clear the liver of any issues such as the presence of too many toxins.

- Andrenal Issues. If a person has high levels of cortisol, there may be a problem with the thyroid hormones' conversion process. Cortisol is a steroid hormone that is released within the adrenal gland in response to stress and low blood-glucose concentration. So if a person is too stressed out, he may have issues with his T4 to T3 conversion as well.

- Medications. Some medications can also affect the conversion process. The most common of these are beta blockers such as the Propranolol which can inhibit the T4 to T3 conversion.

Sample Case: Patient: Janet, forty-one-year-old, married

Issue: Weight gain, inability to lose weight, other issues such as acne breakouts.

Condition: Based on her records, Janet claims to only consume healthy foods and undergo exercises. Her diet was generally clean but she has a tendency to eat more carbohydrate-rich foods than she should.

She is also fond of drinking coffee, which contains impurities that cause inflammation and absorption of more toxins.

Her diet also consists of a lot of meat products. While she refrains from common carbohydrate sources, she compensates her sugar intake by drinking fruit juices instead of sodas.

Her idea of exercise is walking inside a zoo three times a week. For it to be considered an effective exercise routine, the intensity level of walking should elevate the heart rate.

Test Results: Janet's thyroid hormone T3 levels were extremely low at almost below normal values. Her overweight scale is at seventy-five percent and her intestinal ecology test showed a huge yeast overgrowth with low levels of good bacteria. This means she is consuming too much sugary foods that feed the yeast in her gut.

Treatment: She underwent detox. Because most of the T4 conversion to T3 happens in the liver, a person with an unhealthy one might need to undergo detoxification after eating a wide variety of foods that may contain toxins.

I also gave her medical foods and specific supplements to fix her gut issues. The supplements were recommended to ensure that the body gets the necessary nutrients. In some cases, general probiotics can be used to treat similar cases but most of the time gut ecology issues will require supplementing a more specific type of bacterium.

Janet's diet was also changed, focusing more on removing high intake of fruit juices and limiting her carbs. Since most bad bacteria in the body require sugar to thrive and multiply, cutting back on sugar sources can help eradicate them.

She was also advised to convert to a gluten-free diet. Gluten, a mixture of proteins found in wheat and related grains, including barley, rye, oat, and all their species and hybrids, has been found to cause intestinal permeability. It is also known to trigger specific reactions from cells in the gut that causes them to unravel, thereby allowing more substances such as toxins to pass through.

In terms of exercise, she was put on interval training which has been found to help speed up metabolism. Interval training requires a patient to alternately do exercises with different rates of speed or degrees of effort. Janet was asked to begin walking for a short period, then progress into a full sprint for a short distance to suddenly increase the heart rate. It makes the cells produce protein faster and function better.

Results: After a fourteen-day detox, she started to lose weight. She lost five pounds. However, a true detox is not a weight loss program. Losing weight is merely a side effect. After six months under the above stated program, Janet lost twenty-tree pounds. It also fixed her skin problems and she was able to eat a lot of the carbs she wanted after her thyroid hormone conversion was fixed.

Points to Remember:

- The thyroid gland controls a person's metabolic processes.

- It works with the pituitary gland to maintain balance in hormones so that the cells in the body get enough stimulation.

- Most of the time, weight gain is caused by issues with the thyroid gland or hormones conversion.

- When checking for problems with the thyroid's hormones, make sure to undergo testing for all of them to determine what the real problem is.

- Wrong Diet and lack of exercise are not the only factors for weight gain.

- An imbalance in the intestinal ecology can cause severe weight gain.

- Obesity is not an incurable disease. It is a condition that resulted from unhealthy lifestyle and thyroid issues.

Food in Our Life

Food plays an essential role in our lives and affects us tremendously every day. It provides us with the energy we need and vital nutrients needed to help us grow and develop a healthy body. Food is what keeps us alive and active with our everyday activities.

There are different nutrients needed by the body. They are protein, fat, carbohydrates, vitamins and minerals and almost all of them are derived from our daily intake of foods.

Protein plays a crucial role in maintaining and repairing our muscles, skin and bones, blood, and other tissues and organs within our body.

Fat is a secondary source of energy and is stored in our body as a reserve. It is difficult to burn and provides more energy than any of the other nutrients. A good source of fat is milk, cheese, some meat, avocados, nuts, butter and oils.

Carbohydrates are either sugar or starches. Foods that are high in starch are rice, wheat, potatoes and maize while foods that are rich in sugar are milk chocolate bars, honey, fruits and sweets.

Vitamins and Minerals are also called micronutrients and are needed by the body in small amounts but important for good health. These micronutrients also control many actions and processes inside our body.

Aside from the different nutrients needed by our body, we also need the help of fiber and water for a good healthy diet. They are necessary to maintain a healthy diet.

Food evolution

Our early ancestors didn't eat food for pleasure. They were compelled to search and gather foods in order to survive the rugged terrains of their surroundings. Early human ancestors were not in stable houses as what we have now, but rather, moved from one place to another in search for a better source of food. These people typically lived in small groups and were led by people who had the ability to persuade others. Early human civilization generally lived a good life because there was plenty of food around, but they lacked the essential technology needed and could only carry tools that they could bring along with them from various places.

People back then learned to eat insects which as we know now are good sources of protein. No, I'm not asking you to eat insects. They hunted animal meat for food and searched bushes to get berries and other fruits. This is how humans thrived in those days when man was just in search for a better alternative in order to sustain themselves. People had to survive through hunting and searching for bushes and trees that bore edible fruits and berries.

Being omnivorous, meaning both plant and animal eater, has also helped humans to stay at the top of the food chain. We are able to eat meat for protein and plants as a source of other essential nutrients needed by the human body to survive.

The History of Farming

Farming began at around ten-thousand B.C. on the land as we know as the fertile crescent. These early ancestors went to that area in search for food, harvested the wild grains that were growing in that area and found that if they scattered those grains, they could make more food for the tribe. Wheat and barley was first grown at around nine-thousand B.C. in the Fertile Crescent. Wheat became an important evolutionary development in human history. Farming altered the world and allowed human civilization to arise.

Farming allowed early humans to settle in one place and stop being nomadic. It also allowed people to live in larger groups because the technology allowed farmers to grow enough food to support the entire settlement. Therefore, it suggested that people could do some other kinds of jobs. This led to the rise of additional technology which was extremely beneficial to mankind. Societies grew and culture emerged from the early settlements. Government was also established to take control of the surplus food which made them powerful.

The importance of discovering wheat farming

Wheat farming goes back to the cradle of civilization. It was the very first grain to be cultivated for human consumption and became the groundwork for mostly all of our healthy produce around the world.

Wheat is a good energy source. Bread and other foods made of wheat have complex carbohydrates that the body needs. Wheat flour which comes from wheat grains is also an important carrier of vitamins and minerals and is a good source of antioxidants, folic acid and phytochemicals. It has also become a staple food for most people around the world because it can control obesity especially in women. Research has shown that people who eat more whole wheat had considerable weight loss over other subjects. Wheat also improves metabolism and prevents diseases like type II diabetes, gallstones and chronic inflammations.

Environmental changes with farming

The rise of agricultural farming in the world has greatly impacted our environment. Degradation of the environment such as deforestation and over fishing has been a constant aspect of this crisis. It has multiple impacts on other species like habitat loss, soil erosion, pollution and climate change.

Domestication of animals

The domestication of animals played a key part in the development of human evolution. We have a close association with domestic animals throughout our history. Like the early packs of animals who hunted for food, we have patterned our behavior for survival towards what early humans have seen in the animal kingdom.

Domestication of animals can be dated back to early ten-thousand to twelve-thousand years ago. Large animals were domesticated and bred for hunting and gathering food.

Animals have also made resources available for man so that they can live in a land without moving to other places for food. Animals have discharged hard labor in the fields and made transportation easier. Animals are also a good source of fat and protein which improves a person's nutrition.

The spread of animal to human diseases

Zoonotic diseases have plagued humans since time began. Animal diseases are transmitted to humans because of the contact with infected animals. One example is rabies. Although it can be effectively prevented with vaccination, rabies affects the nervous system of a person or mammal bitten by an infected animal.

The great Bubonic plague in Europe was widely caused by a rodent infected with a bacteria and has killed millions of people during the Middle Ages. Salmonella, a common bacterial disease found in foods can also be passed between people and animals. Various animals and pets can carry these infectious bacteria including birds, poultry animals, dogs and even cats.

Farm animals have also carried diseases to humans. Bird flu and swine influenza can be passed on to humans and cause illnesses. Tuberculosis is also one of the diseases passed on to humans. Different animals including cattle and goats carry the tuberculosis bacteria that can carry a lifelong disease. We often become infected if we consume raw or undercooked products from these infected animals.

Genetic modifications of food

Genetically modified or GMO foods first appeared in the late 1990's. Genetically engineered foods are foods made of organisms that have had some changes in their DNA sequence using the science of genetic engineering.

There are several reasons why GMO's are used. Basically, seeds from plants are genetically modified to improve resistance to insects and generate healthy crops. They reduce the risk of crop failure and make crops more resistant to extreme weather conditions.

GMO's are also seen with environmental benefits. They require less chemical, land and machinery, and reduces environmental pollution, soil erosion, and greenhouse gas emissions. Genetically modified foods also are more resilient to infestation because they produce their own insecticides. They also serve for better nutrition. GMO's are produced to contain more vitamin and minerals than the conventional foods we eat.

Though they have beneficial aspects, GMO's also have their downside. They pose a serious allergic reaction to people who are sensitive to certain enhancement chemicals. Genetic enhancement generally incorporates certain proteins not found in the original organism. This can cause allergic reactions to some people. Some GMO's can also lower a person's resistance to antibiotics because they have a built-in antibiotic element by which eating them can diminish the effectiveness of actual antibiotics.

Some common genetically modified foods

There are some common genetically modified foods. They don't appear to be different from the conventional type of food that you see but are genetically altered to be different.

- Corn. The US is the largest producer of corn in the world and corn is a common component of the customary food, landscape, and industrial chemicals. Corn also appears to be the most genetically modified crop. Although they are not intended for human consumption, the biggest threat is that these transgenic corn contaminate the unmodified ones.

- Tomatoes. They are known to be the first widely genetically modified food in the U.S. An enzyme known as polygalacturonase was deactivated to suspend the tomato from rotting. They are then fully ripened on the vine and still lasts longer in the grocery stores.

- Rice. Rice is also one of the most genetically modified foods. It is the staple food of almost half of the world's population. They are modified to make them more resistant to pests and some are enriched with vitamins and mineral traces than the normal rice.

- Milk. One of the most questioned GM foods is the rBGH or recombinant bovine growth hormone. The hormone is amalgamated from genetically modified bacteria which yields higher production of milk by preserving milk-producing cells and keeping them alive inside the cow for a longer period of time. They are mainly criticized because cows are susceptible to diseases and antibiotics given to them would trickle down into the milk supply.

- Potatoes. Genetically modified potatoes are grown and disposed as starch potatoes. Though they lag behind in terms of human consumption, they are processed with foods containing potato starch.

How food becomes extra weight

The main concept here is when you don't burn it off, it stays around in your fat cells. If you need to lose weight, don't eat too many of any one thing and exercise systematically. All of us should know that exorbitant eating leads to excessive weight.

What happens with the body is when the food enters your mouth, your saliva which contains enzymes breaks down the starch in the food and turns it into sugar. This, together with any fat and water in the food you ate, travels to your stomach where it ferments them.

An enzyme that digests protein, called pepsin, and hydrochloric acid works to break down the food and turns it into a substance called chyme. The mixture of chyme and acid goes into the duodenum, the gallbladder secretes bile, dissolving the fat in water, refining it, and making it easier to absorb. Enzymes from the pancreas go into the duodenum to supplement the break down of fat, sugar, and protein. The food is now turned into fluid form and is absorbed by the lining of the small intestines. This is where fat, sugar, and protein go their separate ways.

The sugar component of the mixture goes directly to the blood stream, and a handful of organs take in the sugar they need as it travels through the blood. Part of it is stored in the liver as glycogen, a substance collected in the tissues as a store of carbohydrates. Everything that is left is converted and stored in fat cells.

Digested fats go first to the bloodstream and travels to the liver. The liver burns some of the fat, modifies some to other substances like cholesterol and delivers the remaining to the fat cells, where they stay until they are required.

Protein is broken down into shorter building blocks, known as peptides. They are then further broken down into smaller units known as amino acids. Amino acids are absorbed in the linings of the small intestine and enters the bloodstream. Some of the amino acids build the body's protein reserve while excess amino acids are excreted, and any excess calories from protein that are built up are stored as body fat.

What happens during and after digestion is a small concept. Anything excessively taken is stored as body fat, no matter what you eat. The body only dispels whatever it needs and stores whatever it can't use and turns them into fat cells.

Overeating

Overeating is a compulsive disorder wherein people use food as a way of coping with negative emotions. People who tend to gravitate towards overeating sometimes feel that their eating is out of control and as a result they oftentimes feel embarrassed, guilty or depressed. There are certain reasons why a person could overeat.

- Comfort eating - People who tend to eat more because of improper needs or feelings, to comfort or soothe themselves and tell themselves that they can't exist without them. These people bury their real needs for acceptance, comfort, and attachment. Overeating becomes a way to escape those feelings and typically becomes a reason for wanting foods loaded with fats and sugar. Foods like ice cream or pizza also transfix certain neurotransmitters in the brain, which causes us to feel good at the beginning. But, we get seized by the craving cycles and we crave more.

- Resentment or frustrations - When things do not go the way we want them, our emotions flare up towards others, ourselves or in food. Eventually, we look for something that would ratify our feelings and unfortunately for some, they are bent on seeking out food.

- Suppression of feelings - When we don't want the sense of what we are feeling and we are afraid that we can't handle them, we tend to hide them from ourselves and gravitate towards eating. When a person feels vulnerable, the brain shifts to self-protection mode which is why we often feel inclined to look for something that would soothe us.

- Destructive self-criticism - When things do not go the way we want them or if things go wrong, we have the tendency to blame, to judge and be angry at ourselves. We have the propensity to blame ourselves for everything that goes wrong in our lives and for everything that does not comply with our ideas on how conditions should work. We drift towards overeating because we know it will make us feel worse and out of control.

Brain process of compulsive overeating

The important thing to understand is overeating is just like any problem. It has a solution and can be treated. Your brain controls everything and certain chemical reactions in your brain start up with certain habits that you do.

The brain can be divided into three parts. The thinking brain or neocortex, the midbrain or emotive brain, and the rewards brain (cortico-basal ganglia-thalamic loop). All three parts play a role in keeping your thinking process at work all the time.

What the neocortex does is you know exactly what to do in order to get there. For example, slimming down. The neocortex knows that you have to do some physical activities in order to achieve that goal, but your body does not do anything when the time comes. You keep doing the same thing you do every day because your subconscious tells you what your body has memorized doing. They run automatically, whether it be emotional reactions, attitudes, perceptions, beliefs or feelings. This simply means that when you choose to change a habit, you have a five percent fighting chance against nighty-five percent of who you are.

The midbrain is the part of the brain that deals with emotions. It is the primitive mammal brain or the feeling part of the brain. Two things can happen to the midbrain. The thinking process might make it seem like you'll miss out on this disapproved food more than others or you may miss on the powerful stimuli to sense elation towards the forbidden food. The sense of missing out is where you get an emotional attachment. Contrarily, the sense of elation can make you more vulnerable to becoming addicted to it.

The rewards center is responsible for the compulsive and automatic reactions towards something. The brain is driven towards the promise of a reward. This part of the brain involves your association centers and autonomic conditioned responses. Studies have proven that there is a severe stress feedback when your basal brain recognizes the existence of an object that you desire. So your compulsion sets in, to briefly rid yourself of the unpleasant discomfort associated with the craving.

Techniques to overcome overeating

There are several ways to beat overeating. For most of them, you can change whatever you have the capacity to change. Do whatever you can to lower the feeling of frustration. However, if you cannot change the situation, look for alternatives. Initially, frustration is an overwhelming wave of emotion, the first goal is to ride that wave without binge eating. When you have overcome the intensity, acknowledge the frustration. Create room for yourself so you can move out of the emotions. Then move towards an activity that would utilize the leftover energy. And finally, practice acceptance for yourself. You can cry if you have to. It has been shown that crying removes toxins through the tears and is a way of cleansing the body. After that, you can move forward and start to feel good about yourself.

You can also change how you see yourself. First of all, you have to understand why you have to change. It could be that you are at the outset of having health problems. You need to make a decision about yourself and not let bad things happen. Then redefine who you want to be and how you perceive yourself. Take the negative things about yourself and make them positive. You can always find inspiration in people who have been in the same situation as you are. Make them your positive role models. Visualize yourself as who you want to be. And never ever put yourself down. Create positive statements about yourself and make yourself feel good all the time.

You can also find ways to reset your body to its original state. Detoxification is a way to cleanse your body of impurities. It puts your organs at rest through fasting and stimulates the liver to drive toxins out from your body. Detoxification also improves blood circulation and refuels the body with healthy nutrients.

Food – The Skinny and Fat

In this chapter, we will be talking about your healthy food options. First of all, let us define and classify the different types of food we eat.

Carbohydrates

Carbs are basically molecules that our bodies need for energy. Your body breaks them down into sugar, which is then converted into energy. There are two types of carbohydrates: the simple and the complex.

The Simple Carbs

This type is not very good for your body. They are the ones that get stored in your adipose tissue for energy. As a side note, we should not think that we should totally eliminate fat from the body. Aside from storing energy in the form of fat, your adipose tissue also provides cushion and insulation to the body.

However, we do need to regulate simple carb intake, especially if we lead a sedentary lifestyle. The problem is that we eat too many carbs and do not move enough to use them up. Thus, the amount that your body doesn't need is stored as fat. This nasty habit of consuming too many carbs than is good for you causes your adipose tissue to expand and expand, making you get fatter and fatter.

Simple carbs include junk food, soda, candy, fruit juice (loaded with high fructose corn syrup), and basically all other manufactured or processed food such as pasta, bread, pizza, peanut butter and other spreads.

Junk Food

The term 'junk food' is in itself quite self-explanatory. These have a disturbingly high content of calories from sugar or fat, but with little or no protein, fiber, vitamins or minerals. In other words, they provide empty calories, having no nutritional value and are ultimately stored as fat. The funny thing is that manufacturers are now 'fortifying' chips with vitamins and minerals, so that consumers feel less guilt about buying their products. Small amounts of certain nutrients are indeed added, but the fact remains that eating a bag of these chips still give you loads of salt, sugar, hydrogenated oils, MSG, maltodextrin and other chemicals we can't even pronounce. The amount of 'junk' can never be truly balanced or somehow justified simply by adding a few milligrams of Vitamin A or whatever. In every bag of unhealthy chips, the potential damage far outweighs the minute good that was added simply to somehow appease the guilt of the consumers.

Sweetened Soda

Soda water is actually good for the body. Aside from rehydrating your body just as well as plain water, it also has been found to improve overall digestion and gallbladder health, as well as prevent constipation. On the other hand, its sweetened and flavored counterparts are very destructive to your overall health and well-being. They are loaded with sugar, or other sweeteners that are even worse than sugar. Believe it or not, a can of soda has ten teaspoons of sugar! Sugar, along with citric acid, has acidogenic and carcinogenic potential. In addition, it also erodes the enamel and creates cavities. Colas, in particular, contain phosphorus that eliminates calcium through the kidneys, resulting in low bone mineral density. While plain soda water will not add extra fat, the flavored ones usually have sodium, all sorts of sweeteners and flavors, acids and other additives. Each of these ingredients may have hidden calories, plus more sodium than your body requires. Here's what you should basically know about carbonated drinks.

- Club soda has sodium, while seltzer water does not.

- Tonic water is high in added sweeteners and flavoring.

- Flavored sparkling water usually contains citric acid and other sweeteners, plus a load of sodium and caffeine.

Soda water adds zest to otherwise plain water, which can sometimes be difficult to drink. To encourage children and adults alike to drink plenty of water and keep hydrated, try adding slices of fresh fruit, such as lemon or apple, and honey to a glass of plain soda water. You may also benefit from adding some herbs and spices such as ginger root or tulsi (holy basil) leaf, cucumber and aloe vera, which are good for the body.

White Pasta

Another thing you should avoid is pasta. Most people think they're doing right by opting for a bowl of pasta instead of the regular burger. And so they sit down in a restaurant and eat a bowl of pasta, which is about four or five cups and more or less three-thousand calories. For a hundred-eighty-pound male who exercises on a regular basis, two-thousand calories a day is okay. The rule of thumb is that a person should consume ten calories per pound of his or her body weight. But if you're eating three-thousand calories in one meal, with negative nutritional value, then what is that bowl of pasta doing to your body? Your body can only use and burn up some of it. The rest will be stored as fat. So that single bowl of pasta is equal to a month of going to the gym. That's how you quantify it.

White Bread

White bread is the modern bread. Unfortunately, white flour is actually bad for your health. It is highly processed, bleached and most probably genetically modified. Bread today is also high in sugar content, aside from it being already high in calories from fat.

Now there are a lot of bread companies that claim to be the healthier option by labeling their bread with 'whole wheat.' But it's just another marketing ploy, a sham. This 'whole wheat bread' is, in reality, simply made of wheat that has been dyed in order to appear like whole wheat. You're not only eating white flour; you're also eating dye. As unfortunate as it can be, colored bread is what passes as whole wheat nowadays. These unscrupulous manufacturers even sprinkle oats or some grains on top of the bread to make it look healthy and hearty. You probably think that you're eating healthy bread but when you read the ingredients, it's mostly sugar. The really infuriating thing about this is that manufacturers are not honest in their labeling. This applies not only to bread, but to almost all other food products as well.

You see, manufacturers are required to list their ingredients from the biggest down to the smallest amount. Knowing that consumers are now more concerned about their health and carefully read the ingredients, manufacturers list different names of sugar in their label. For instance, you might read: "wheat flour, hydrogenated vegetable oil, sugar, buttermilk flavor, high fructose corn syrup, milk powder, glucose, dough improver, sucralose, etc." Sugar, high fructose corn syrup, glucose and sucralose are all forms of sugar. And they divided the total sugar content of the product into these different names, so as to somehow mislead people. If they simply put 'sugar,' that will be the first on the ingredient list. And with this high sugar content, people will have to think twice before buying their product.

Ideally, you should stay away from white bread as much as possible. Unless you're in Western Europe, in Holland or Germany for instance, then healthy bread is well within reach. The bread they have there is almost black or dark brown in color and is really thick and hard. They do not make use of yeast, improvers, softeners or other chemicals in their bread. It's almost like eating grains. It's hearty and delicious. If you can find that kind of bread in the US, then lucky you! However, the possibility is highly unlikely. Now, if you're used to eating white bread, then you're going to have to learn eating healthy bread, which can be hard. It can be categorized as an acquired taste. Not many people can appreciate it, but it is great for your body.

Commercial Peanut Butter

Peanut butter and jelly is probably your kids' favorite lunch. One piece of white bread is usually accompanied with a tablespoon of jelly and a teaspoon of peanut butter. For lunch, we usually give our kids two pieces of this. Unknowingly, we are slowly but surely feeding our children with poison. Here are the hard facts about peanut butter.

To make it creamy, flour and hydrogenated oil are added. Plus, the jelly is high in sugar content. It's basically candy. That's why kids love it. The white bread is high in sugar. The peanut butter is high in sugar. And the jelly is high in sugar. On a regular basis, we are giving our children lollipops, ice cream, peanut butter sandwiches and whatnot. No wonder kids today are obese and diabetic. Unknowingly, we are feeding our loved ones with sugar on top of sugar. In reality, we are actually pawns that play a big part in developing a diabetic nation. So if you really think about it, you're feeding your kids a 'diabetes' sandwich. Add to that lunch pack a bottle of fruit juice, which is not pure fruit juice at all but mostly sugar.

On the other hand, if it's pure, unsweetened peanut butter, then it is high in protein. Here's a tip. When you go shopping for peanut butter, choose one with oil floating on top. It's a good indication that it's natural. Just mix it. The ones that look good and have great-looking texture are filled with hydrogenated oils, homogenizers, stabilizers and so on. Also, stay away from the ones that have too many ingredients. It would be best if you choose a peanut butter with basically two ingredients: peanuts and salt. Now if you look at the big brands of peanut butter, they have perhaps twenty ingredients and the second on their list of ingredients is sugar. In the US, most companies mislead people by labeling products with 'no added sugar.' It's a bit tricky really. "No sugar added" implies that it has no sugar content, but what it actually means is that there is no extra sugar added. What makes it even worse is that it has high fructose corn syrup, which is even worse than sugar.

Let me share with you my personal experience with peanut butter. Before I knew what eating healthy was, I used to think eating a peanut butter sandwich was healthy. But as I became more educated, and as I started to truly understand what a carb was, what a protein was and what fat was, I started to look at different options. I tried eating real peanut butter but didn't like it because it tasted a bit bitter. Anyway, let's fast-forward to a couple of years. I started to understand the need for detoxifying, fasting and resetting everything. After my detox, I decided to start again with the peanut butter. This time I was able to taste the sweetness in the peanut butter. While before, it tasted horrible. The point is, your taste buds can change and adapt. If you're reading this book, I want you to understand that all this is attainable. It's not at all far-fetched. In due time, you will actually start enjoying some of the things you didn't think you liked in the beginning. And you can start by detoxing and resetting your taste buds to their normal and natural mode.

Here's another trick in controlling your food intake: Eat for your health, and not simply for your tongue. As a matter of fact, it is one of the principles of yoga, wherein you are taught to control your tongue and eat only what is necessary for the health and maintenance of the body. We should control the tongue, instead of letting the tongue control us. In the truest sense, we should eat to live and not live to eat.

The Complex Carbs

This type of carbohydrate is broken down by the body into sugars as well, but it has less of an insulin spike. Insulin is what's released by your body (your pancreas in particular) in response to the food you eat. As food is broken down into sugar and into different saccharides, they are pushed into the muscles and into the fat cells with the aid of insulin. In other words, insulin prevents your body from releasing fats out of the cells so they stay stored.

Complex carbs are also rich in fiber, which has the following benefits:

- Fiber helps lower your blood cholesterol levels and thus reduces the risk of heart problems.

- It alleviates constipation and other gastrointestinal issues.

- It aids in controlling weight. With foods high in fiber, you will almost immediately feel full and satiated with fewer calories.

- It also helps control diabetes as it slows down the entry of sugar into the blood.

Moreover, complex carbs also do not have much glycemic load, so the body does not necessarily need to store them in the adipose tissue. On the contrary, they are used up by the body right away. Vegetables are a great source of complex carbohydrates.

The Vegetarian Diet

The vegetarian diet, or at least a diet consisting mostly of vegetables, is great for your health. Not only are vegetables rich in complex carbs, they are also rich in vitamins, minerals and a ton of nutrients good for the thyroid. Minerals from the soil are absorbed by these plants. And when we eat them, we get a good supply of these minerals. Not only that, we also get a lot of water. Water makes up much of the fruits and veggies we eat. In fact, there are animals that depend solely on fruits and veggies, and these are where they mainly get their water. Also, in emergency cases, if you get stranded on an island, you can live on coconuts. You won't believe how wonderful coconuts are for your health.

The Tree of Life

With a thick, impenetrable shell and husk, the coconut water inside is clean, pure and rich in electrolytes for rehydration. A lot of athletes are now drinking this. In Asian countries, the white coconut meat is also utilized. In the Philippines, for instance, it has been the olden Filipino way to grate the coconut meat and squeeze it to extract the coconut milk. This coconut milk is then used in many native dishes and sweet delicacies not only in the Philippines but also in other neighboring countries. Today, vegans are now resorting to coconut milk as a substitute for cow's milk. They even use it to make vegan chocolate and ice cream.

While on the subject of coconuts, let me tell you a few important things about coconut oil. Now, there are some sources that say that coconut oil is bad for you. But this is not true. The problem is that we have so many different sources that tell us what's good for us and what's not, and it can get confusing. Even reputable sources, such as WebMD, are saying that coconut oil is not good for you.

But coconut oil is really good for you. It's one of the best oils you can get. It's a medium-chain triglyceride, which is immediately used by your body for energy. You don't have to worry about insulin spikes or that it will make you fat, because it will be immediately used up by the body.

So, you have to be very careful and not believe right away something you read on the internet, no matter how reputable the site may be. You have to read the research yourself. I highly recommend that you start taking a teaspoon of virgin coconut oil a day. It will do wonders for your overall gut health. Your digestion and elimination will become smoother and more regular because of its high fiber content. Being a medium chain triglycerides, coconut oil goes from your digestive tract and straight to your liver. Here it is used as an instant source of energy. Specifically, they are turned into ketone bodies, which have positive therapeutic effects on brain disorders, i.e. Alzheimer's and epilepsy.

Going Natural, Fresh and Organic

Leading a healthier lifestyle and opting for a greener diet can be tricky. What with all the genetic modification, not to mention the use of preservatives and other chemicals for longer shelf life, fruits and vegetables today are available in supermarkets even when they're not in season. Most of us try to be vegetarian to be healthier but eat canned fruits and vegetables marinated in brine or syrup, plus a load of other chemicals.

Here are a few tips to get the most out of vegetables.

- It would be best to eat vegetables that are in season. It is Mother Nature's arrangement that certain fruits are grown at certain times of the year to sustain your specific body needs for that specific season.

- Eat organic ones you can buy in the farmers markets. They're all natural and not genetically modified.

- Stick to fresh produce. Stay away from canned and frozen fruits and veggies.

Healthy Food Suggestions

To help regulate your blood sugar and blood pressure levels, as well as to control your glycemic and insulin index, we recommend that you eat more of these:

- Brown, red and other unpolished, unbleached and organic rice

- Whole grains

- Beans

- Vegetables

- Fruits

- Greek Yogurt

It would be best if your start inculcating good eating habits in your kids while young, so they can follow this as adults and keep obesity at bay.

Choose to Be Wise

We should understand that most magazines and blogs use only clinical studies to promote whatever it is that they want to push. Politics and marketing have one thing in common. According to the agenda they want to push, they will release certain claims and studies. So when some site says that something is good for you, you should suspect it's probably sponsored by some company. Someone's always going to pay. Look at the lobby for cigarettes. They said cigarettes were good for you, that they aid in digestion, etc. Big tobacco companies claim that there is no study proving that cigarette smoking is bad for your health. However, there are a good number of studies showing that cigarette smoking is bad, and perhaps only one or two show it is good for you because they paid for it.

We must not easily believe what we read. The scientific method of thinking should always be applied in every aspect of life. Make the necessary research and follow the weight of the evidence. After all, your health and the health of your loved ones are on the line here.

Carbohydrates are sugars, fibers, and starches found commonly in all the foods we eat. Though often rejected in weight loss diets, carbohydrates, one of the most basic food groups, is necessary for a healthy life.

Carbohydrates are macronutrients and are one of the main ways the body receives energy or calories. It is the body's main source of energy. We just need to know that there are good carbs; complex carbs. They are termed carbohydrates because at a chemical level they are molecularly composed of carbon, hydrogen, and oxygen.

There are three main types of macronutrients—carbohydrates, proteins, and fats. Macronutrients are important for appropriate body functioning and the body has a need for large amounts of them. All these types of essential macronutrients are only obtained through the foods we eat as the body cannot create them on their own.

The recommended daily allowance for carbohydrates in an adult is a hundred-thirty-five-grams, however, people are advised to have their own personal carbohydrate goals as people with varying age, build, and daily activities depend on how much their intake of carbs is.

Carb absorption for most people should be between twenty five to forty percent of the entire calories. One gram of carbs is equivalent to about four calories, therefore a diet of a thousand-eight-hundred calories a day would be equivalent to about one hundred twelve grams at the bottom end and 180 grams of carbohydrates at the top end. It is advised though for diabetic people not to eat more than two-hundred-grams of carbohydrates per day.

Benefits of carbohydrates to our body

Too much carbohydrate intake is the first reason to be pointed out when someone gains weight. While some people think that reducing carbohydrate rich foods intake will do much to lose weight, it is important to know that not all carbs are bad for the body. Carbohydrates, for a fact, if chosen precisely, not only reduce weight but can have many other health benefits.

Carbs mainly fuel the body with energy. Simple activities like breathing requires the use of energy and the main source of the body's energy requirement comes from glucose. Glucose is derived from the sugars and starches that you eat and is broken down into simple sugar in the process of digestion. Insulin is main ingredient used to store glucose in the body. After the process, they enter the cell walls and any extra sugar circulating in the blood is stored in major body parts such as muscles and the liver, and is then converted into fats.

Carbs can also help with controlling weight problems. They are most often seen as the main cause of being overweight, but choosing the right carbohydrates can help you reduce or control your weight. A good selection of fruits, vegetables, and fibrous foods are likely to be helpful in controlling weight and managing muscle tone unlike what is being heavily advertised by popular diet regimens.

The important function of carbohydrates

Carbohydrates mainly add fuel to the central nervous system, provides power, and energy to working muscles. They are also used primarily by our body to prevent the usage of protein as an energy source. Carbohydrates also enable fat metabolism and play a significant role in brain function, including mood management and memory. Carbohydrates are also a fast energy source. The recommended daily amount of carbohydrates is established on the amount of carbs the brain requires to function.

Types of carbohydrates

There are two classifications of carbohydrates, they are the simple and complex carbohydrates. The only difference between the two types lies in their chemical composition and how immediately they are digested and absorbed by the body.

Simple carbohydrates are easier and are more quickly absorbed by the body. They primarily consist of one or two sugars, namely fructose, commonly found in fruits and lactose, found in dairy products. These single sugars are also called monosaccharides. Carbohydrates from sucrose or table sugar, lactose from dairy products, and maltose found in some vegetables and beer are called disaccharides.

Simple sugar can also be found in most candies, refined sugar, and syrup but they do not contain essential vitamins, minerals, and fiber. These forms of simple sugar are also called empty calories and lead to weight gain. Simple sugar gives you a burst of energy because of the faster rate that they are digested and absorbed. They lead to spikes in blood sugar levels and can give a person what is known as a sugar high.

Complex carbohydrates are composed of long chains of simple carbs, usually three or more simple carbs linked together. They are also called polysaccharides and are often referred to as starchy foods. Complex carbohydrate food contains vitamins, minerals and antioxidants. Foods such as green vegetables, brown rice, oatmeal, quinoa, and beans are good examples of foods with complex carbohydrates. They usually take time to be digested, broken down by the digestive system and absorbed in the body.

Good carbohydrates vs bad carbohydrates

Carbohydrates are found in most food that we eat. Some of them are good for your health such as vegetables while others like donuts are perceived to be composed of bad carbohydrates. Commonly known foods which are recognized as bad carbohydrates include processed foods, sodas, white bread and all those that often do not contain any nutritive value.

Bad carbohydrates usually are high in calories, contain a lot of refined sugar, has highly refined grains, low in nutrients and fiber, high in sodium and may sometimes contain saturated fats, cholesterol and trans fat.

Complex carbohydrates are found in foods such as whole grains, vegetables, fruits, beans and legumes. They may contain low to moderate calories, have high nutritive value, low in sodium, saturated fats and trans fats, and does not contain refined sugar and grains.

The effects of too much or too little carbohydrates on our body

When we eat food containing carbohydrates, our digestive system digests the food and breaks it down into sugar. The sugar then enters the blood and as the blood sugar level rises, the pancreas secretes insulin, a type of hormone that stimulates cells to absorb the sugar either for storage or for energy. As the cells absorb the sugar in the blood, the sugar levels in the bloodstream start to drop. When the process begins, the pancreas starts producing a hormone called glucagon to signal the liver to initiate the release of stored sugar. The exchange of insulin and glucagon sees to it the that the cells everywhere around the body, including the brain, have a constant steady supply of blood sugar.

Carbohydrate metabolism plays a significant role in the increased development of Type II Diabetes. This happens when the body cannot produce enough supply of insulin or cannot properly utilize the insulin the body creates.

Type II Diabetes gradually progresses over the years, when initially, the cells and other muscles cease to respond to the hormone, insulin. This status, known as insulin resistance, roots from blood sugar and insulin staying at high levels despite the time taken after the process of digestion. As the time progresses, the heavy requirements made on the insulin-making cells eventually wears them out and the production of insulin ultimately ceases.

Hypoglycemia is also a cause of not getting enough carbohydrates in the body. If you are not getting enough supply of fuel, the body has no energy to dispense. In addition, with the lack of sufficient glucose, the central nervous system's function deteriorates, and leads to the feeling of dizziness, physical and mental weakness.

When people experience hypoglycemia, the body will use protein as its energy source. This can cause problems to the body as the body needs protein to build muscles. Using protein as a replacement for carbohydrate energy takes its toll on the kidneys, which leads to painful passage of byproducts in the urine. Additionally, people who suffer from not getting enough carbohydrates have a deficiency in fiber, which leads to digestive problems and constipation.

The significant role of insulin in metabolism

Insulin is a hormone secreted by the pancreas which allows your body to use glucose taken from carbohydrates in the foods you eat to either use as energy or store it for future use. Insulin plays a vital role in keeping your blood sugar level stable from not getting too high or what is known as hyperglycemia, or getting too low which is called as hypoglycemia.

The cells inside our body require sugar for energy. Anyhow, sugar in the blood cannot go directly into most of your cells after eating food. When this happens, the beta cells inside your pancreas create a signal to discharge insulin in the bloodstream. Insulin then affixes itself to other cells so that the sugar is absorbed from the blood. Insulin plays a crucial role to unlock the cells and to give way for the absorption of the sugar into the cell to be used for energy.

If you have more sugar in the body than what is required, insulin supports the liver in the storage of excess sugar in the body. It also aids in the release of the hormone glucagon when the body requires the need for sugar such as during physical activities and in between meals. Consequently, insulin aids the body to balance blood sugar levels and control them at a normal range. When the blood sugar level ascends, the pancreas does the role of secreting more insulin. If your body does not create enough insulin to support the absorption of sugar, or your cells become resistant to insulin, you can possibly develop high blood sugar, which over time can cause serious complications as your sugar levels in the bloodstream elevate for a longer duration of time.

Some misleading food label pitfalls to avoid

Food companies recognize that health or the appearance of health is marketable, but some labels can be misleading. Research has shown that phrases like organic tend to make people believe that the food they are buying is low in calories or high in protein even though the food may be highly processed with lots of sugar and high in calories. Although these labels may be factually right, they create a broad feeling towards what they actually contain.

The tabbed banner of nutritional facts embellished on the frontal part of different products or what is known as the Facts Up Front is created by the food industry. If you look it up, you will see certain numbers for saturated fats, calories, sodium and sugar besides nutrients to reassure and encourage people to buy them. Several proclaimed health products laud their health benefits when they contain added sugar and other unhealthy benefits. Manufacturers also use vague descriptions like "Helps Support Immunity!", to depict how a single food component may alter the function of a body part. That can be ambiguous and deceitful. Such claims tend to be just marketing strategies and may commonly have high sugar or sodium content and saturated fats.

A lot of people are also inclined to look at products with the phrase "high in fiber". These products may be high in fiber because they contain detached fibers in the form of purified powder like maltodextrin. These form of fiber do not have the same valuable health effects as those found in vegetables and fruits.

Food manufacturers also use phrases like "made with whole grains". These type of labels do not guarantee that the product is mainly or predominantly made from whole grains. They might even contain just a trace of whole grain components and may be loaded with sugar and calories.

Another pitfall to take notice of is the small portions of the serving sizes. The tiny servings create an impression for making unhealthy substances look less bad. An example would be that one serving can contain a certain amount of calories when in fact a person can eat the whole can and thus get much more than what he thought he was gaining.

Five Super Healthy High Carb Foods

Carbohydrates are wrongfully blamed for the obesity epidemic. However, the fact is not all carbs are created equal. Highly processed foods are sugary and mostly composed of refined grains which are clearly unhealthy and fattening. However, it does not go with fiber-rich foods that additionally contains carbohydrates. Here are some of the high-carb vegetarian foods that are especially healthy.

- Quinoa. Quinoa is a protein rich food that contains twice as much fiber as most alternative grains. It is also rich in vitamins and minerals such as iron, lysine, magnesium, manganese and Vitamin B2. Quinoa is also classified as a pseudo cereal, a seed that is prepared and ingested like grain. It has been associated with health benefits like better blood sugar control. Quinoa is gluten free which makes it a popular alternative to those who are gluten intolerant.

- Oats. Oats are known as the healthiest whole grain food on earth. It is a good source of mostly all vitamins, minerals and antioxidants. Raw oat has an average of sixty-six percent carbohydrates and has a high fiber content. They are exceptionally high in a potent soluble fiber called beta-glucan, a form of sugar found in the cell walls of plants such as oats and barley. Beta-glucans are commonly used to reduce the risk for high cholesterol, diabetes, cancer, and HIV/AIDS.

- Buckwheat. Buckwheat is greatly nutritious and consists of more antioxidants and minerals than most grains. Eating buckwheat is beneficial to heart health and blood glucose control.

- Bananas. Bananas contain about twenty-three percent carbohydrates in the forms of starches and sugars. Green and unripe bananas have more starch which eventually turns into sugar as they ripen and turn yellow. They contain good plant compounds and are high in potassium, Vitamin C, and Vitamin B6. Bananas are good for lowering blood pressure and beneficial to heart health. Unripe bananas also have resistant starch and pectin, good for digestion.

- Sweet Potatoes. Natural sweet potatoes are a good source of Vitamin A, Vitamin C, and potassium. They have a high antioxidant content and contain up to twenty-one percent carbohydrates. They also are a rich source of starch, sugar, and fiber.

Food choices that increase your risk for diabetes and other diseases

There are certain food groups in our modern day diet that greatly increases our risk for developing type II diabetes. It is extremely important to know which of these inhibit the risk of contracting the debilitating disease. Aside from a genetic disorder, there are certain food groups that are known possibly to cause the disease. They are:

- Highly Processed Carbohydrates. These foods are manufactured and void of important healthy nutrients like vitamins and minerals. They do not contain fiber which is helpful with digestion. Most of these products are easy to digest and can cause a spike in blood sugar and insulin levels. They are the primary culprits that needs to be eliminated as much as possible. Highly processed carbohydrates like pasta, crackers, cakes, bread and a variety of products available in the market must be consumed in moderation to reduce the risk of diabetes.

- Sweetened Drinks. Sweetened drinks contain excessive calories which most often leads to weight gain. Insulin resistance can also be a common possibility, from consumption of these

126

drinks, because of too much sugar load. Sweetened drinks include beverages like sodas, sweetened fruit drinks, sweet teas and a multitude of different products that are main causes of high glucose levels. One way to eliminate this in your diet is to drink more water instead to be hydrated. It is also advisable to avoid putting too much sugar and cream in your coffee or tea.

- Processed & Red Meat. Processed meats have been closely linked to type II diabetes. Studies have shown that an eighty-five grams serving per day of red meat can greatly increase your risk for type II diabetes to almost twenty percent. A small amount of processed meat can increase your risk by up to fifty percent. Replacing them with other healthier sources of protein will reduce your risk for heart diseases and diabetes. You can have sardines, organic poultry, or salmon instead and eat it with a lot of vegetables. It would be a much healthier alternative.

- Saturated and Trans Fats. These fatty oils are loaded in almost all of the modern products that we eat. Trans fats are found in baked and fried foods predominantly in restaurants. Saturated fats are those found in some butters, fatty meats, full milk and cheese. To ward off saturated fats, try to cook your food with avocado or olive oil. You can also choose lean meat and avoid skins from poultry, dress your salads with vinegar or lemons instead of choosing heavy dressings.

Ethnic food suggestions for a healthy meal

Greek yogurt. Greek yogurt, nonfat or low-fat are good additions to a healthy meal. They are low in calories and are loaded with live bacterial cultures. Greek yogurt is strained largely to take out much of the liquid whey, lactose and sugar which gives it a thick consistency. It is also doubly packed with protein while the sugar content is cut in half and is high in protein. Greek yogurt is popular among vegetarians as they contain the needed protein identical to that of lean meat.

Ceviche. Ceviche is a packed with lots of Protein, Omega-3 Fatty acids, Vitamin B12 and Phosphorus. It is a food native to Latin Americans made of fresh fish marinated in citrus juice and mixed with other variety of ingredients such as onions, tomatoes and bell pepper.

Mediterranean Greek Salads. These type of salads mostly contain vegetables which are a great source of vitamins and minerals. A toss up of spring mix Mediterranean salad contains romaine lettuce which is good for the skin and bones. Sun Dried tomatoes are high in alpha-lipoic acid, lycopene and other essential vitamins good for the heart. Added ingredients like feta cheese which is a good source of calcium keeps the bones strong. Balsamic vinaigrette helps improve digestion and immunity.

Guacamole. Guacamole is made from ripe avocados mixed with garlic and fresh tomatoes, onion, cilantro and lime juice. They add an exciting flavor to meals and have essential nutrients that are healthy for your body. Guacamole has unsaturated fats which lowers damaging blood cholesterol and lowers blood pressure. It has Vitamin C, good for the skin and strengthens blood vessels, and Vitamin E which slows down oxidative damage to cells.

For someone who has a problem with weight maintenance, it is crucial to know how many food calories you take in every day. It is important to know whether your body is taking in the exact amount of calories needed by the body and to avoid excessive calorie intake.

A calorie is literally a unit of energy. We get the calories from the foods we eat daily, which is needed to fuel our body with the energy we need to do all our activities. All foods have a distinctive calorie amount content. Fats, a natural greasy substance found in animal bodies, has the highest concentration of calories. It contains nine calories per gram of pure fat. Carbohydrates and protein each contain the same amount-four calories per gram of pure protein or carbohydrate.

Knowing and understanding how many calories a certain food contains helps you balance your calorie intake and help manage your weight regulation goals. To retain a stable weight, the amount of energy we put in our bodies must be the same as the amount of energy we expel during bodily functions and physical activities. If you put in more calories in a day and store more energy, there should be a balance of activity to maintain a balanced weight.

Gaining excessive weight happens when we put in more energy than what is needed by the body. It then stores it over time and becomes body fat. Studies have shown that almost all adults eat and drink more than the body needs and have the tendency to think that they are more physically active than the truth. This in turn, leads to health complications over time.

How to calculate your daily calorie requirements?

The body's calorie requirement depends upon a few factors. Among them are your age, height, gender and the level of daily activity. Calorie intake also depends on whether you are trying to lose, maintain or gain weight.

The number of calories one takes in also depends on the size of the person's body. Usually, large people require more calories than smaller people. A person's daily activity also has to do with the amount of calories he needs every day. Men generally require more calories than women do.

The natural human system uses about sixty percent of calories in keeping up with its natural processes at rest. It is computed as what is called as the Basal Metabolic Rate or BMR. The leaner muscles a person has, the higher your BMR. By building lean muscles, you boost your body's calorie burning abilities.

The rest of the calorie index is divided between any bodily activity and digestion. A body requires thirty percent of calories for any physical activity whilst, ten percent of it goes to the process of digestion. In this sense, it is imperative to eat smaller meals a day more often as digestion burns more calories in the process.

There are several formulas for determining the BMR of a person. They do require personal information such as the weight of the person, the height, and the age.

To compute for the BMR of an average American male, the equation is (12.7x height in inches) + (6.23 x weight in pounds) - (6.8 x age) then add 66 to the total of the BMR. For the average American woman, the equation is (4.7 x height in inches) + (4.35 x weight in pounds) - (4.7 x age). Then add 655 to the total of the BMR.

Meal Frequency and How Much to Eat

Eating smaller meals every two to three hours has been found to boost metabolism. It is better than big, infrequent meals a day. Foods that are high in protein and fiber are essentially beneficial to the body as they pack in more vitamins and minerals needed in digestion and bodily functions. Ultimately, with the many debates about whether to take in as many meals a day or fewer, it all boils down to the caloric intake of your body, the types of calories, and knowing how many calories a certain food has and how much of it is needed by your body to achieve and maintain the amount of weight that you want.

Studies have also found that parents have a big impact on children and how they eat as they grow into adulthood. Researchers have found that children who eat with their parents during mealtime tended to eat more fruits, dairy products, and vegetables than those who didn't share meals with their parents. These children are drawn to eat nutritious foods than their counterparts. It also plays a role in developing a healthy and well-adjusted child who has high self-esteem and improved academic achievements.

Unhealthy Foods High in Calories

While it is common to spot an unhealthy food high in calories. There are several out in the market that we commonly consume. Among those are the following list:

- Fast Food Meals. Normally, most fast-food served meals are mass-produced, highly engineered, and have very low nutritional value. They are relatively cheap but on the health aspect can cost you twice the value.

- Sugary Drinks. This is the most common content for our modern diet. It is seen as the most fattening agent of our diets. When we take in these sugar calories, the brain does not register them as food. For this reason, a person's tendency is to compensate by drastically eating

133

more calorie loaded foods instead. Sugar though, when consumed in large amounts, drives insulin resistance in the body and is heavily linked to the non-alcoholic fatty liver disease.

- Ice Cream. Ice cream is considered one of the most delicious foods in the planet but is loaded with high calorie content and is easy to eat exaggerated amounts. Taking it in as a dessert after a meal makes it even worse as it adds up to your total calorie intake.

- Processed meat. Processed meat has been closely linked to serious diseases such as colon cancer, heart ailments and type II diabetes. Opting for healthier choices of unprocessed meats which does not contain a lot of unhealthy ingredients would be better to keep your calories in check.

- High-calorie coffee drinks. Coffee is commonly high in antioxidants. Studies have proven that people who drink coffee have lower risk of contracting serious diseases like type II diabetes and Parkinson's. However, some cafes have turned them into unhealthy beverages with empty calories, and lots of artificial sugar and cream which are not good for your health.

Healthy Foods High in Calories

There are also several foods that are healthy and high in calories. This is essential if you are looking to gain weight or to maintain the current weight that you have.

- Eggs. Eggs are a good source of high quality calories and protein, half of which is concentrated in the egg white. They contain almost every nutrient we need and also have trace minerals along with other major vitamins and minerals essential in maintaining a healthy body. They also raise the High Density Lipoprotein or good cholesterol in our body and lowers the risk of heart diseases and other health problems.

- Avocados. Avocados are an abundant source of nutrients. Along with that, they also come with a hundred-and-sixty calories and seven grams of fiber. Also known as alligator pears, avocados are loaded with essential fats, and various other important nutrients like vitamin C, K, and E.

- Dark Chocolate. These sweets are rich in fiber, Iron, Magnesium, Manganese and other minerals. Several researchers have found that they also lower the risk of heart diseases and can improve overall health. Dark chocolate made of cocoa has a hundred-and-seventy calories per one oz. of serving.

- Fresh fruit juices. Fresh fruits and vegetable juices can have high caloric content. Prune juice has up to ninety calorie content and grape juice has seventy-six calories. They are also a good source of vitamins and minerals and have no fat content. Fruits and vegetables also have low energy density, which means you can eat a lot without loading too much on calories. They are good proponents of weight loss - eating lesser calories but feeling full and gratified.

- Peanut butter. Peanut butter has five-hundred-eighty-eight calories per one hundred grams. They are good for weight maintenance because they digest slowly which leaves you with a feeling of fullness. Peanut butter is a good source of protein, phosphorus, vitamin E and other essential vitamins.

Healthy Eating Habits

Having healthy eating habits is a way of maintaining a good and harmonious relationship with yourself. There are several ways to achieve this. One way is not to give up everything. This helps because being too strict on yourself will eventually have a rebound effect by overeating if you are not satisfied. Getting a small amount of the things you love will make you feel less deprived of the good things that you enjoy and thus, will not lead you to crave for those things.

It is also important to always have a plan. Don't get thrown into the lure of a good looking restaurant menu when you are hungry. You don't even have to be strict with what you would like, but always see to it that you maintain a balance of everything. If you have to go heavy for breakfast with potatoes and meat. Go easy on them for lunch. Make sure to have a balance of healthy fruits, vegetables and snacks for the rest of the day. In fact, it's best practice to eat breakfast like a king, lunch like a prince and dinner like a pauper.

You don't have to eat boring food all the time. You can spice up your vegetables and fruits by adding some complimentary taste to them. Adding some high-flavors can prep up your taste buds to looking forward to nutritious foods. Try adding some salt and pepper or tomato sauce to a plain cooked vegetable to make them taste more palatable.

You can also spend more time preparing the foods yourself. Studies have been found that people who spend time preparing their foods correlates to improved and better eating habits. These people who spend time purchasing, washing and preparing them right away tended to use their vegetables more so than those who didn't. Otherwise, it's chips and dips.

Choosing fruits and vegetable that are colorful equips your body with good phytonutrients which are needed for the body to fight diseases. Choosing vegetables and fruits that are colorful will help the body raise the amount of vitamins, minerals and other plant compounds essential to keep the body strong and resilient.

Research has also found that people tend to make the wrong choices when they are in the midst of hunger after doing something which requires more energy. People tend to turn to high calorie foods in order to satisfy their need for more energy. Choosing alternative snack treats like yogurt or nuts can be helpful if you are trying to maintain or lose some weight. It will satisfy your cravings without sacrificing the need for too many calories in your body.

Good food intervals

The most efficient way of losing weight is to spread your meals steadily throughout the day. In this way, there is an even balance of carbohydrates, protein, fats and other micronutrients in your diet. Eating smaller meals a day will stimulate your metabolism and prohibit you from getting hungry. The ideal time for each meal is no more than four hours a day, with the exception of sleeping hours. Falling off short of taking meals frequently will slow down your metabolism and will make you more likely to overeat during mealtime.

Breakfast

It is highly suggested to never skip breakfast because it turns on your metabolism for the day. Skipping breakfast can make an impression of starvation on your body and will most likely slow down your metabolism to conserve energy. Eat meals that have a high concentration of complex carbohydrates and protein such as eggs and fruit or any food that will give you energy all day will be helpful in keeping you energized. Also, remember to eat the largest amount of your daily calories at breakfast. This causes your body to expend more energy.

Lunch

Lunch is also an important meal to keep your metabolism ignited throughout the day. Choose meals which are high in fiber, have complex carbohydrates and protein.

If you have no time to prepare your own food, you can look for a deli which serves foods with lots of vegetables. Or you can choose to have Greek salad, with lots of tomatoes, cucumber and olive oil, good for the heart. Getting a good load of protein, which takes longer to digest will keep you going all day long. Sandwiches made of whole grain, vegetables and lean meat like turkey is also a good choice.

Dinner

Dinner should be the last and smallest meal of the day. Take in something that can be easily digested by the stomach. You can eat a small meal as you won't need that extra energy because you will just be sleeping. A small meal of whole grains, fruits and vegetables will suffice to give you the energy you need all night.

Snacks

Snacks can be inserted in between meals. You can take them before each major meal time within the day. A healthy snack made of fiber, protein and fat will delay digestion and supply a solid and stable release of energy.

Eating something starchy or sweet will give off a burst of energy which will leave you fatigued within the hour. Choose something that is light but will give extra energy to keep you going and not leave you feeling famished.

To make your mealtimes less boring, you can also change your eating patterns every now and then. Instead of eating cereal during breakfast, which we often do, you can eat them during dinner. After all, who decided which foods to eat for breakfast and dinner. Eating this way makes your meal more interesting and less of the conventional way. You can also choose foods that are more appetizing and naturally colorful giving you more vitamins, minerals and phytonutrients needed by the body.

Fiber and its significant role

Fiber is the part of a fruit or vegetable that is not easily digested by our digestive system. There are two varieties of fiber. Soluble fibers turn into gel in our stomach, slows down digestion and makes us feel full. It helps cut down serum cholesterol and blood sugar in the blood.

Insoluble fiber though has an important role of helping the body move the food we eat through the digestive tract. It remains unchanged in form throughout the digestion process and makes the waste product heavier and softer so it goes smoothly out of our body. Fiber also adds to our body's protection towards diseases.

Fiber or dietary fiber found in food is important nutrient needed for proper digestion of the foods we eat, efficient function of the digestive tract, and helps us feel full. A deficiency in fiber leads to complications like colon cancer, constipation, elevated levels of cholesterol and glucose in the blood, and hemorrhoids others.

There are foods that contain high quantities of good fiber. Common superfoods such as cereal contains 5 grams of fiber, oatmeal contains one-point-seven grams per one-hundred-grams. Avocados are also a rich source of fiber containing six-point-seven grams per half if eaten raw.

Some useful tips for people who do not cook at home

Cooking can be a way too complicated task for anyone. Mixing all the ingredients, how and which goes first becomes a tricky situation. Cooking might not be for everyone, but in order to have a healthy life, we must have healthy choices with the foods we eat.

If you are one of those people who find it hard to cook for yourself or your family, there are ways to get those vital nutrients in the body without making those failed efforts. One of them is to make smoothies out of vegetables and fruits. It is one of the quickest and easiest ways to ensure that you get all those vitamins and minerals found only in them. All you need is a blender, a mixture of fruits or vegetables, water and any other healthy ingredients you might want to add, blend it for a couple of minutes and wallah you have a healthy drink.

The recommended daily allowance for an average American is two cups of fruit per day, it might be an apple or banana depending on your choice and three cups of raw or cooked vegetables. There are a lot of choices to choose from and it all depends on what you like.

You can also make sandwiches for yourself or your family. Sandwiches are easy to make and do not require cooking. Make sandwiches that have a lot of vegetables in them like lettuce and tomatoes, add in some unprocessed cheese and toss in a slice of unprocessed meat. It makes for a complete package of carbohydrates, protein, vitamins and minerals.

If you don't have enough time to go through all of this, you can simply choose a deli that offers healthier choices of foods. They may not be hard to find around your area, it's just requires going out of the way and starting to look for these places. They may be quite pricey compared to some of the local ones, but in the long run they are all worth it in terms of a healthier choice.

Some tips

- Change what you want. If you are not eating more than you need but still not getting the desired weight, the problem might be the choices you make with the foods that you eat. Changing what you want and getting all the nutrients that your body needs will suffice to keep you grounded with your weight. Learn to know what is right and make those choices for you.

- Fix your body first. Fixing your body first will ultimately keep you at bay from having problems with yourself. Having meals at the right time and improving your metabolism goes a long way to fix any problems that you may have with your weight. Knowing what is right and what to avoid will also do good to keep you in tune with your body.

- Remove emotional ties with food problems. Emotional eating is a way for some people to remove stress and reward themselves rather than satisfying hunger. This becomes a way for some people to make themselves feel better towards something. It is important to know that emotional hunger or emptiness is not a means to fill hunger. It may be an underlying psychological problem that needs help in some way.

How to Treat Thyroid Problems

By not taking good care of your body, your thyroid can suffer from two forms of illnesses—hypothyroidism and hyperthyroidism. These are diagnosed by knowing the amount of thyroid-stimulating hormones (TSH) that are produced in your body. TSH is the chemical produced by your pituitary gland that helps thyroid release its own hormones such as the thyroxine (T4) and the triiodothyronine (T3). Both thyroid hormones play crucial roles in stimulating your body's metabolism. You can go back to Chapter 4: The Thyroid, to refresh your knowledge on this topic.

Hypothyroidism is typically diagnosed when there is a high amount of TSH in your blood while the thyroid is releasing low amounts of thyroid hormones. Hyperthyroidism on the other hand, is when there is an insufficient quantity of TSH and the thyroid releases more hormones.

Warning signs that your thyroid is not working

You might have seen drastic changes in your body such as weight gain, low immune system, and fatigue over the past

146

months and may not know the causes of these changes. A malfunctioning thyroid can be the problem. Aside from weight gain, below are several signs that you should be visiting an endocrinologist immediately.

1. **Inability to focus**. Your mental activity can be affected if you have a weak or malfunctioning thyroid. You often experience memory loss, indecision, mental fogginess, and an inability to concentrate on a certain task. High or low levels of thyroid hormones will result in sluggishness and depression, which will eventually affect the alertness of your mind.

2. **Mood changes.** Your change of moods can be drastic. From a depressed to an extra jubilant state. Your energy level can also be extreme at some point. You will go from strong and active to lethargic in a few minutes.

3. **Dehydration.** People with thyroid problems often experience mild to extreme dehydration. In fact, it is one of the causes of an underactive thyroid gland.

4. **Muscle cramps and pain.** If you have not been doing strenuous activities lately but are feeling muscle fatigue and pain, have your thyroid checked for any abnormality.

5. **Intolerance to heat and cold.** People with overactive thyroid glands become easily irritated

with heat and in areas having high temperatures. On the other hand, those with an under-functioning thyroid system cannot take cold and winter seasons. They often feel cold.

6. **High pulse rate.** Palpitations are one of the major signs of hyperthyroidism.

7. **Menstrual changes.** If you are suffering from long and excessive monthly bleeding, you could be experiencing hypothyroidism. Conversely, if you bleed less than normal and have shorter menstrual days, you could be experiencing hyperthyroidism.

In these cases, if you are having a hard time losing weight and feeling most of these symptoms, you may want to visit your doctor immediately to address possible thyroid issues.

Causes

Your thyroid fails when your body is not healthy or is experiencing imbalances due to adjusting your lifestyle, diet, and daily activities. Like a car that needs to be maintained regularly, the body also needs to be in its best shape at all times. Aside from having an unhealthy lifestyle, these factors can also be underlying causes of your thyroid problem:

1. **Autoimmune disease.** This happens when your own body produces antibodies that work against your tissue. Instead of protecting you from

infections and diseases, it is the one attacking you. Doctors are yet to discover the reason for this betrayal behavior of the body, but few presumptions say that a virus or any element that is alien to the body is causing the action.

2. **Radiation.** If you have been exposed to radiation, it could trigger hypothyroidism.

3. **Thyroidectomy.** Through surgery, portions, if not all of your thyroid gland can be removed. This, in turn, will result in the cessation of thyroid hormone released by your thyroid.

How to know if you have a problem with your thyroid?

There are different ways to find out if your thyroid is healthy or if it is suffering from hypothyroidism or hyperthyroidism. One is performing a radioactive iodide uptake tests. This method determines the amount of iodide that is in your thyroid.

If you do not consume the required amount of iodide your body needs or you have too much of it in your gland, you will be at risk for thyroid problems at some point in your life. Iodine, or potassium iodide is responsible for keeping your thyroid gland in its best shape and function. Thus, by looking at your iodide content, doctors can easily see

Weight… It Might Be your Thyroid – Dr. Michael Scott

whether or not you are suffering from a thyroid problem.

The doctor will have to put a device over your neck area and you will have to consume a radioactive iodide solution to gauge the radioactivity level of your thyroid gland. This method will be repeated a few more times to gather more information. If the results show that you have high amounts of iodide, the doctor will then run a radioactive iodide uptake scan. This step will show which part of your thyroid gland is producing large volumes of iodide. It will also show the gravity and the condition of your thyroid. Has the iodide been spread evenly or unevenly in your tissues? Are there any nodules in your thyroid area? And if yes, are they the culprit for the unwanted hormones? If the nodules are in fact the culprit for the excess hormones, you may have hyperthyroidism.

Nodules could also become cancer. If the doctor sees that it has a potential to turn into cancer, the patient will have to undergo a blood test and/or biopsy or Fine Needle Aspiration. Through fine needle aspiration, a sample will be collected by inserting a needle into the affected area or an area where there seem to have lumps and abnormalities. Lumps, cysts, nodules, and enlarged lymph nodes can be discovered through imaging tests or by pressing the area. Determining if there are any abnormalities in your thyroid is the first step to treat the said health issue so you won't be

150

barking up the wrong tree.

Before undergoing fine needle aspiration, you should not take aspirin or any other blood-thinning medicines. Your stomach should also be empty hours before the test—no food or water.

Things can get crazy with your thyroid gland; thus, a regular checkup is a must.

What can I do to treat my thyroid?

There are two ways to treat thyroid problems—through over-the-counter medicines and through changing your lifestyle and diet. Both are effective, but to keep your thyroid healthy throughout your life, a complete lifestyle change is a must.

Below are ten ways to treat your thyroid condition using both alternative and conventional treatments.

Conventional and surgical approach:

1. **Radioactive iodide treatment.** This is a form of radiotherapy that treats thyroid cancer. If your thyroid problem has gotten this severe, then this is one of most effective options to cure the problem.

2. **Anti-thyroid drugs.** Also known as thionamides, these anti-thyroid medicines can treat hyperthyroidism. Examples of these drugs are methimazole or propylthiouracil. These can be used before you undergo radioactive iodide treatment or thyroid operation. These are also important in reducing your chances of undergoing such treatments.

3. **Surgery.** Your doctor may use this procedure to remove part of or the entire thyroid gland.

Alternative treatments:

A very effective way to treat thyroid problems is to follow a healthy lifestyle. Here are seven ways to treat your thyroid and prevent thyroid problems naturally.

1. **Reduce your sugar and caffeine intake.** Sugar and caffeine are the number one enemy of the thyroid gland. From flour to fruit, the body treats them as sugar. This doesn't mean that you should be eliminating these foods from your diet. The secret is to choose wisely and plan your meals. Forget about soda and beer; rather, choose real fruit juice with no added sugar. And this means that you may have to make your own beverages. Yes, it'll take some time, but in return, you will enjoy your years without having to suffer thyroid disease and its symptoms.

2. **Increase your protein.** If you are a meat-eater, upping your protein is not a big deal. Same goes with vegans and vegetarians. There are many food sources that are high in protein, which by the way, produce more protein than red meat and eggs. These are nuts, quinoa, legumes, soy, and soy products.

3. **Consume good fat.** Getting rid of all the fats in your body is a crazy idea, because your body needs fat. Imbalance in fat can affect your thyroid. Good fats include fish, nuts, butter, cheese, yogurt and coconut products.

4. **Supply your body with vitamins and nutrients that are lacking from your diet.** Your diet may be lacking from a particular nutrient your body needs. Take multivitamins to supplement your body's optimum requirement.

5. **Avoid gluten.** Gluten can be a major culprit as to why the body is building up antibodies against its own tissues. This is because the thyroid gland has a similar molecular composition as gluten. The body will treat the thyroid gland as if it is gluten thereby producing antibodies that attack your thyroid gland.

6. **Improve your gastrointestinal tract.** Your thyroid is dependent on the condition of your gut; thus, if this organ weakens, or is in imbalance you can expect to suffer thyroid problems.

7. **Get rid of stress.** Thyroid is a sensitive gland and is very receptive to all kinds of stressors—be it

emotional, physical, or mental. So practice activities that can kick stressors out of your system such as yoga and meditation. Embrace the outdoors and get full body rest.

Motivation

In the previous chapters, I have shared with you some very basic and important knowledge about your body and how you can scientifically and safely transform it into a better and healthier shape. However, knowledge alone is not enough. You have learned so much already about how to effectively lose weight, but may still end up not implementing these practices. Why? It's could simply be the lack of creating a motivational environment. I, for instance, have done my part in imparting these crucial pieces of information about your thyroid and how to safely lose weight. But it will be up to you to create an environment that helps you actually follow and apply what I have shared in this book. Motivation is necessary to follow the program. In fact, motivation is the key to succeed in any endeavor.

As your doctor and well wisher, allow me to leave you with a few important points to remember to keep you motivated throughout this program.

Give It a Chance, One Last Chance.

I know you're tired, frustrated and heart-broken. Your self-esteem has been shattered into smithereens and you're thinking: "Hey, perhaps it's time to give up and accept that

I'll be overweight for life." You regularly go to the gym four or even five times a week, eat a healthy diet and restrict calories, you've been fanatically following this routine for two or three years already, yet still can't seem to lose weight. You've tried everything in your power and capacity to lose weight but without any positive result.

You may even have gone to your primary care doctor with hopes of getting help for your unexplained weight gain and impossible weight loss despite all austerities and sacrifices, and all you hear is suspicion and doubt suggesting you're not really following a strict diet and exercise regimen. I know it can be disheartening when people, especially your own doctor and family, don't believe you *are* eating right and exercising like crazy. But please don't give up just yet. Give this book, this program, one last chance. See this as your last card, a wild card if you must. Besides, the most that is asked of you is to set three minutes a day, three days a week of exercise to speed up your metabolism and effectively shed those otherwise stubborn pounds. The rest of the program involves only very minor lifestyle changes and temporary mineral supplementation.

Knowledge is Power

Knowing that there is a real answer and solution to your weight problem can be enough to motivate you. Now, you're no longer as hopeless as you were before. You have found out that the reason behind your weight loss failures may be purely biological. Keep in mind the knowledge and real-life cases I've shared with you in this book. The goal is achievable. Losing weight is truly obtainable. All you need is a little science, a shimmer of hope and an adequate amount of motivation.

With the patients I've treated, I've seen their self-esteem boost back up, and it's truly fulfilling. It's heartwarming that these persons, who have been frustrated and depressed due to their weight, have ultimately ditched their multiple anti-depressant medications and have become their *regular* selves again. It's almost like rebirth, or winning the lottery. There's sheer elation and joy for life. It seems like a dark cloud has been lifted and they are enjoying life in a fresh and new light. And I simply am out of words to describe how I feel that the simple knowledge that I've shared was able to have that big of an effect on people's outlook, their well-being and their lives in general.

Give Up the Blame Game

It's not your fault. No, it's really not. So stop punishing yourself for something in your body that you have no control over. As a matter of fact, around twenty million Americans suffer from thyroid diseases in one form or another. Not everyone may understand that you're not losing weight due to *biological reasons*. But you and I *do*. Together, we can effectively counteract this discrepancy in your body, the safe and healthy way. When you walk across the street and start feeling paranoid that people are staring and whispering about your size and about how careless a person you are for letting your body gain that much weight, remind yourself that it's not your fault *at all*.

Exercise and calorie restriction can be useless if the reason is biological. It's not important if other people don't know about this biological reason behind your physical condition. What matters most is that you know it and I, your doctor, know it. You have no obligation to prove to people, whom you don't even know, that it's all biological. Forget about them, and focus on *us* and *our program*. If you do, the results will prove themselves without any need for your explanation or justification. It's your body and not theirs. Simply try to stick to the program and all will be well.

Stop Comparing Yourself with Others

No two persons are born equal. Not even identical twins. This we must understand and keep in mind. No one has the exact same set of fingerprints as yours. In other words, each and every one of us is unique, not only on the external physical aspect but more importantly on the internal physical aspect. Even identical twins who share the same genetic code have different fingerprints. Over time, they will also grow up with differences in their physique and overall health, depending on their environment, diet and habits. One twin may be physically fit and healthy while the other might be obese. No two persons can ever be exactly the same, so there's no point comparing yourself to and trying to be better than the person next to you. There's a thin and almost invisible line between looking up to someone for motivation and looking at someone for envious comparison and competition. You deserve to be a better version of yourself, and not of anyone else.

Determine Your Motivation

It is intrinsic human nature to be narcissistic or selfish. And this trait is making itself even more manifest and overtly obvious in the form of 'selfies.' People are documenting their lives moment by moment via Facebook, Instagram or other social media sites. And for most people, this selfie trend is one form of motivation for weight loss. Everyone wants to look great and take that perfect selfie shot. By regularly taking selfies, whether you upload them or not, you are somehow documenting and comparing your past and current body size. If you're an already active social media kind of person, then it wouldn't hurt if you make good use of your selfie addiction for keeping motivated.

On the other hand, if you're a more conservative type of person, then you can find other ways to keep motivated. First, determine the reason behind your desire to lose weight. If it's not out of a purely selfish motive, then lucky you! You have a great chance of staying motivated. Why? Because if you're inspiration is your child or your aging mother, then you are most likely to stick to your austerities.

Weight… It Might Be your Thyroid – Dr. Michael Scott

You want to stay fit and healthy not just for the sake of looking great, but also feeling great and functioning to your maximum physical potential for the sake of your loved ones.

I would say that, indeed, love is the best motivation for anything, even for weight loss. If you wish to lose weight and be fitter and healthier because you want to be able to take care of your aging parents or to be able to see and hold your future grandchildren, then that's the best motivation you can get. Selfless motivation, if I may personally say so, is more stable, more fruitful and more fulfilling than a selfish one.

Here's my personal tip: Place photos of your loved ones by the mirror, the refrigerator, your treadmill, or anywhere you exercise. It's a good reminder that you wish to be healthier to be there with the ones you love, for longer. To take things a step further, simply devote a few hours each week for outdoor playtime with your kids (biking at the park or playing Frisbee on the beach) and set a regular and feasible exercise routine with your husband or wife (jogging together at the bay walk or on the beach three times a week). With the active involvement of the most important people in your life, then you are more compelled to achieve your goal.

Step Out of Your Comfort Zone but Don't Push Yourself Beyond Breaking Point

The cliché 'No pain, no gain' is relatively true. You will have to make the necessary sacrifices and undergo some change if you truly wish to succeed in losing weight. However, you shouldn't strain yourself beyond your personal limits.

Here's another tip for keeping your motivation levels stable: Understand that motivation levels naturally fluctuate. It's like fuel in your car; it naturally runs out. But you can still drive and reach your destination even without having a full tank all the way. All you need to worry about is preventing it from running empty. Some days you will have better motivation than others. You shouldn't focus too much on this or unnecessarily worry about it. You can't just externally and superficially keep your motivation level to the roof all the time. That would be almost impossible and draining. When you feel that your motivation starts to wane, take the necessary break. After two to three days of rest, introspect and ask yourself the following questions:

If I give up now, what will I see in the mirror six months or a year later?

If I give up now, how will I feel in those coming months?

Weight... It Might Be your Thyroid – Dr. Michael Scott

If I give up now, what will happen to my health?

If I give up now, what will be the effect on my friends, family and loved ones?

Take breaks but don't give up. Besides, all you are asked to follow is a three-minute exercise a day for three days each week to help boost your metabolism. Add to that routine the healthy diet suggested in this book and the supplement/s to be prescribed after the necessary tests, and you're on your way to a fitter and healthier you.

An Advice to Women (And to men who love their wives, girlfriends, sisters and daughters)

As mentioned earlier in this book, people suffering from hypothyroidism are easily fatigued and irritable, gain weight rapidly and have sleep problems—symptoms that are also linked with depression.

To my female readers, please note that, statistically, you are five to eight times more prone to suffer from thyroid issues than your male counterparts. In addition, diagnoses of depression are also found to be more common in you than in men. This is mainly due to biology. Again, it's not your fault. The spells of depression you undergo on a constant basis are most often hormone-induced.

This is quite observable and obvious during the pre-menstrual period. Due to your fluctuating levels of estrogen and other hormones before and during the menstrual period, you experience these depression-linked symptoms. In fact, all throughout your life, your hormones will continue to fluctuate, not only before and during menstruation, but also during pregnancy, after child birth and around your menopausal stage. Of course, symptoms vary from one woman to another but generally, these hormonal irregularities will cause fatigue, disturbed sleep, weight gain and changes in skin. And oh yeah, mood swings. You can't miss that one, for sure.

So what's the point? My point in reminding you of these obvious facts is this: Accept and understand that you are bound by these biological inevitabilities. There's no escaping them, unless you are one of the lucky ones who have but only mild pre-menstrual issues, no post-partum blues or depression and moderate menopausal symptoms. Most women have to deal with such issues on a monthly basis. And add to that a weight loss program and life becomes chaotic.

Sticking to a program is already difficult in itself. If you're a woman with constant hormonal fluctuations, mood swings and short spells of depression, then sticking to a weight loss program can prove to be quite a handful.

Here's my advice: anticipate these regular spells but do not wallow in them. It will be hard but try to keep in mind that it *will* pass, and that you should stick to the program no matter what. It's just your hormones; they should not define you.

Better yet, you can follow this program with the help of other women in your life who would undoubtedly understand each and every step in your healthy body transformation. Women should be able to understand other women better. Your girl friends or your sisters can prove to be your best motivators in achieving the fit and healthy body you desire.

Find a Role Model

Super-skinny models are not recommended as effective role models. So you'd better not pin or post photos of such persons on your bedroom wall, as they do not really serve as a good inspiration. In fact, looking up to them can potentially hurt your progress. Other doctors claim that such images can be discouraging to women, as they create highly unrealistic self-standards. And I agree. You should never compare yourself to these super thin models. In fact, unfortunate as it can be, most of these super-skinny girls suffer from eating disorders and are underweight. Or, in real life their figures may not be as perfect as shown in magazines but have really been airbrushed and manipulated by Photoshop.

Here's what I recommend for you to do instead. To stay inspired and motivated, post images of yourself at your healthiest weight. Remember how it felt when you could still do the things you now find impossible to do, like riding a bike or playing tag with your kids, or whatever inspiring memory you may find. Hold on to that feeling and memory to keep your motivation stable and steady. Or you can look at photos of real men and women before and after their weight loss journey for added inspiration. That's how you keep things real and obtainable.

Don't Rely Too Much on What You See in the Mirror but on How You Feel

We often experience frustration when we focus on a specific number on the scale. In other words, our fixation on our visual senses is not a healthy way to keep motivated. Standing in front of the mirror or checking the scales more often than necessary actually does more bad than good. It's also a sign of impatience. Stepping on the scale once a week or every two weeks should be sufficient. Keep in mind, however, that as your body adjusts to your new regimen you may gain a couple pounds in the first thirty days. Don't panic! As your body adapts the weight will begin to come off continuously.

Instead of looking and looking, you should become more attentive and sensitive to your body by focusing on the feeling you experience after eating a healthy meal or after each exercise. Hold on to that great feeling. That would be sufficient to sustain and even increase your motivation, even when you're not seeing much changes or results just yet.

Patience truly is a virtue. Remember that your hormones are still regaining their balance. It's not something you can rush. No one loses a significant amount of weight overnight. If someone claims that you will have your desired body weight in two weeks, think twice. More often than not, these drastic weight loss strategies are unsafe, unhealthy and temporary. You may unknowingly be risking your gut health, and exhausting your water and protein reserves instead of the fats. These unscientific weight loss programs are the reason behind your yoyo weight-gain-then-weight-loss cycle. You starve your body for a while, and then it resorts to using up stored water and protein. Then, after this state of starvation, your body will naturally want to replenish itself and so, you start gaining this water/protein weight back with a vengeance.

Just follow the simple diet and exercise recommendations in this book and, one day, once you do look in the mirror, you will be surprised at what you will see.

Don't Be Too Hard On Yourself

Most people make use of self-criticism to somehow motivate themselves to lose weight. However, this actually does more harm than good. Once you enter a self-critical mode, you engage the portion of your brain that is associated with your fight-flight survival reflex. This, in turn, results in an increase in your cortisol ("stress" hormone) levels making you crave sweet and fatty foods.

You will regularly find yourself in spurts of self-criticism and it will be difficult to overlook or ignore them. The best you can do is to bring your consciousness back to the knowledge that it's not your fault that you're overweight. It's biological, and you are already doing your best to stick to the program, speed up your metabolism and lose weight.

Go easy on yourself and regularly remind yourself that you're on the right path. If you contemplate on and wallow in self-criticism or self-pity, visualize the effects these negative feelings will have on your hormones. Think about it. The program we have is for you to bring the balance back to your hormones. You shouldn't let your stress hormones get all riled up and counteract the good effects of our program.

Another thing, instead of sulking over your unwanted weight and the things you cannot do because of it, you should try to be more appreciative of what you *can* do. For instance, you still can walk, move and function normally on a regular basis. You're luckier than the guy who had to be towed out of his own house because of his size and weight. A crane had to be used to break down the walls and tow him out of bed because he could neither fit through the door nor walk. You, on the other hand, have this chance to change your life for the better. Try to appreciate and be thankful for this fact.

You can stick to the program and still have fun. Go out, relax and unwind. Read a good book or watch a movie. Spend time with friends and family as usual. After all, you're still you, whatever size or shape your body may have. The program we suggest is relatively easy, with very minor lifestyle changes that don't involve starving yourself or exercising like crazy. It's really a very practical and sustainable lifestyle that you can follow not just for a couple of months but possibly for the rest of your life.

Liver Health

What is the Liver?

The liver is a large lobed glandular major organ located in the abdomen of vertebrates, along the right side of the belly. Typically, it cannot be felt from outside the body since it is covered (and protected) by the rib cage. It weighs about three pounds, has a rubbery texture and is reddish-brown in color.

It is comprised of two parts known as the lobes, which are separated by a group of connective tissue that also serves as anchors to the abdominal cavity. The right and left lobes are located above the gallbladder, which serves as storage for bile, yellow, brownish or olive green liquid that is also produced by the liver.

Liver is also known for its functions in human metabolism particularly in breaking down proteins into amino acids. But unknown to most, the liver has another important function: it is responsible for the body's detoxification.

Liver as a Filter

The body doesn't need everything that we consume. This is why we were made with a filter known as the liver. This vital organ filters everything a person eats or drinks and gets rid of those that the body does not need-particularly toxins.

The liver is usually involved in filtering unneeded substances from alcohol as well as medications, which is why people who are alcoholic or who would be taking a strong drug are recommended to test for liver malfunction.

Like any other filters, the human liver has a certain limit. A lint filter, for example, becomes full of lint and therefore, does not function as well as it used to. Another example of a filter that can be compared to the liver is an air-conditioning filter. Over time, it becomes clogged with dust, dirt and other small particles that it has gathered from filtering the air in the room.

When the filter is too clogged, very little or no air comes through the air-conditioning unit. In the same way, when the liver is not cleaned regularly enough, it becomes clogged and does not function as well as it used to. When this occurs, there is a high probability that the toxins gathered in the liver affect the function of the other organs in the body.

The only difference between lint and air-conditioning filters and the liver is that the latter cannot be changed—at least not that easily.

How the Liver Works

The liver is made up of many smaller units known as the lobules. Blood coming from the digestive tract passes through these lobules via a portal vein to the liver. This blood, which is set for filtering carries nutrients as well as medication and toxic substances. Before it proceeds to the rest of the organs, the liver makes sure that the blood has been rid of these toxic substances known as toxins.

After being filtered, the nutrient-carrying blood is processed, detoxified, stored, and altered. After that, the nutrients are then passed back into the blood or released in the bowel to be eliminated, depending on the body's need for it. This is of course a simplified explanation.

As mentioned earlier, the liver is also responsible for producing about eight hundred to one thousand milliliters of bile per day. According to the U.S. National Library of Medicine, bile is necessary for the breakdown and absorption of fats. From the liver, it collected in the small vessels where it is passed to the main bile duct. From there, the substance is carried to the duodenum, a part of the small intestine.

The liver also has an important role in human metabolism. In fact, it can be considered an essential organ for the breakdown of proteins into amino acids. Amino acids in food are then turned into energy to be used by the body. The liver is also responsible in making carbohydrates or fats, leaving a toxic substance called ammonia as a by-product in the process. To make sure the body is not poisoned, the liver converts ammonia into urea, which is released into the blood and transported to the kidneys. There, urea is passed out of the body by means of the urine.

Things That Are Bad for Your Liver

Many people are aware that alcohol has a wide range of negative effects on the liver and yet most of them continue to abuse the depressant drink. Aside from causing malfunction of the liver, alcohol is more popularly known to cause alcoholic cirrhosis.

According to the American Liver Foundation, **alcoholic cirrhosis** is the most advanced type of alcohol induced liver injury. It is characterized by scarring—or the emergence of hard scar tissue that replaces soft healthy tissue. The organization revealed that about ten to twenty percent of all alcoholics, around the world, suffer from alcoholic cirrhosis. Unlike other disease, this condition cannot be reversed by abstinence though refraining from drinking alcohol might help alleviate the symptoms of liver disease and avoid further damage.

Other liver diseases caused by alcohol include hepatitis and fatty liver disease.

Meanwhile, **medications** have various effects on the liver. Unfortunately, many of them are not good.

Some drugs can directly injure the liver as it passes through the organ where it is filtered and broken down. Others affect the liver indirectly or by means of the chemicals they are converted to when the liver has already broken them down. Overdoses of medications like acetaminophen (Tylenol) are known to cause liver disease. This condition is called **dose-dependent toxicity**. There are also cases when drugs can cause **allergy** in the liver characterized by inflammation. The inflammation happens when the immune system attacks the medications.

Weight… It Might Be your Thyroid – Dr. Michael Scott

What is Medical Detox

Every person—it doesn't matter who you are—needs to clean your liver.

Usually used in drug abuse case, medical detoxification is now being tapped as a viable means of ridding the body of many other toxins even if they have not tried illegal substances in their life. Detoxification focuses on the liver but it has other effects that make people want to undergo it: medical detox causes weight loss.

What is NOT Medical Detox

By doing a medical detox, you're allowing your liver to function. Metabolism speeds up because toxins are being removed, other bodily functions work better. But many have repeatedly made the mistake of using cleanses to achieve results that only detox can do.

A cleanse is something that helps remove food that you have stored in your gut. Cleanses are usually characterized by limiting one's diet to juices that are rich in fiber and other non-alcoholic fluids. They are good for ridding your gut of the solids that may have built up but cleanses cannot detoxify your body.

Weight… It Might Be your Thyroid – Dr. Michael Scott

When you cleanse, you lose weight because you deprive your body of food. This is not necessarily beneficial especially if you are not consuming any protein-rich food required for your body's vital processes.

If you are cleansing with a protein-less diet and exercise, your body is eating its own muscle. This is because protein is the body's battery and without it, the body will have to compensate. The weight you lose in this case is muscle, which is actually something you need to really lose weight.

This is why I do not recommend cleansing very much. Special diets with exercise makes one lose muscle, which is actually bad if you want to burn fat. If you wanna do it the right way, it's best to do a medical detox.

There are some products sold in the market that do not really work. These products, or should I say, "propaganda," are meant to "sell to your emotion" and take advantage of a person's dire want for a "quick fix" for weight loss.

In fact, the term detox has been repeatedly misused and turned into a marketing strategy, which treats a nonexistent condition.

Real detoxification isn't ordered from a menu of alternative health treatments, or assembled from ingredients in your pantry. Actual detoxification is provided in hospitals under life-threatening circumstances — usually when there are dangerous levels of drugs, alcohol, or other poisons in the body. Detox kits are not something that can be purchased so easily over the counter of any pharmacy.

Actors, actresses and even fitness experts are often used to advertise most of these products but these faces for hire do not always use the brands they promote. Achieving the same body as a certain celebrity is virtually impossible since they do not have the same genetic makeup as we do. Then there is the matter of knowing these celebrities' entire lifestyle, which plays a big role in a person's weight loss. This is why it is still best for people to be smart when choosing a way to lose weight and learn all about medical detox and how it really works.

What is the Digestive System?

The parts of the digestive system usually referred to as the gut is comprised of the intestines. The digestion process begins in the mouth, then through the stomach and to the intestines.

With around one hundred thirty trillion bacteria in the intestines, there are ten times more cells in the intestines than the other parts of the body. In fact, it is probably one of the longest organs in the human body with a surface area comparable to that of two tennis courts.

The digestive process begins in the mouth where food is chewed and broken down with the help of enzymes from the saliva. Since it is the first phase of digestion, chewing should be taken more seriously. Chewing the food we eat slowly can do miracles for our digestive system and entire body. In fact, it is explained that chewing food very well until it reaches an almost fluid-like consistency makes digestion easier. Plus, it helps prevent us from overeating.

From there, the chewed food proceeds to the stomach where it gets injected with acids from the stomach and the pancreas. Here, the food undergoes another phase of digestion, which entails the food being broken down more into liquid form before it goes to the intestines.

As the food travels through the gut, good bacteria break it down further into small-chain fatty acids and medium chain fatty-acids, which are primarily absorbed through the portal vein during lipid digestion.

The bacteria, which are living organisms working independently but in harmony with our body, draw out the nutrients such as vitamins and minerals from the food we consume. After that, the broken down food nutrients travels through our bloodstream to the liver where toxins are filtered.

Since it is the body's main biochemical synthesizer and detoxifying organ, the liver filters the blood to remove unnecessary substances not only once, but several times. The medical terms "first pass," "second pass," and so on refer to the blood being filtered numerous times in the liver.

Gut Ecology Imbalance

Like Mother Nature, the gut ecology or the so-called intestinal flora as mentioned in Chapter four should maintain a balance. This means there should be enough of a particular bacteria and not too much of another.

If the balance of the intestinal flora is thrown off, there is a great chance that there would be an overgrowth or undergrowth, which leads to the dominance of bad bacteria. This can then lead to several ailments such as inflammatory disorders, chronic headaches, GERD, thyroid disorders, irritable bowel syndrome, constipation and many others.

Many medical practitioners have accepted the common notion that such issues automatically arise when a person has reached a certain age. This belief may be a result of the fact that as people get older and neglect to undergo detox, the gut becomes more permeable to bad bacteria. The fact is, the person's age is not the issue—it is the current state of the body filter, which is the liver that should have been maintained through medical detox regularly.

Parasites in the Gut

A vast majority of us have parasites in our guts. which enter our bodies through the food and beverages we consume. Traditionally, people undergo a medical process to remove parasites regularly and then test for parasites. This is because medical experts know that it is not a question of if the person has a parasite but a matter of how many.

My study revealed that one hundred fifty million children with intestinal parasites are found to have decreased test scores, focus issues and get tired easily. This is because their bodies consume more energy in the digestive process, which should have been instrumental for better mental performance. Aside from that, they were not able to receive the necessary nutrients they need to perform well in these areas because the parasites beat them to it.

The balance in gut ecology can be determined by a stool test. This examination allows medical experts to see the levels of bacteria in the person's gut and determine when there is dysbiosis, or microbial imbalance inside the body.

Balance in the gut ecology is very crucial to human development because it can affect the body's processes. If there is too much or too little of a certain strain of bacteria, the body won't function well. When this happens, the person experiences a number of disorders such as bloating, which is caused by an overgrowth of bacteria in the intestines.

Fortunately, bringing back balance in the gut ecology does not necessarily require intake of many medications that eradicate bacteria altogether. Since killing bacteria does not necessarily solve the problem, I recommend the use of natural supplements and healthy foods to help the body get back to its natural balance. These supplements do not kill bacteria but instead, provide nutrients for existing-but-lacking good bacteria to reproduce. Once the number of the lacking bacteria is up, the balance in the intestinal flora would be restored.

In cases when supplementing the existing bacteria is not enough, I recommend the intake of probiotics, which are actually good bacteria. However, let me emphasize that since there are different kinds of good bacteria, it is important to seek professional help to determine the specific kind of bacteria that is lacking and what probiotic would be able to supplement it.

It is important to repair the gut first before taking any kind of probiotics. Repairing the gut entails fixing the intestinal lining, removing the excessive bad bacteria and inoculating in what's missing in the good bacteria—a process that typically lasts for four to six months.

Case Study: Nancy, eight years' old

Nancy had difficulties concentrating in school, leading her teacher to think she had attention deficit disorder (ADD). She also had plenty of attitude problems and temper issues signified by her short patience especially when she argued with her parents.

Initial Action:

Because of her unruly behavior, Nancy's parents took her to a child psychiatrist. Fortunately, the doctor also happened to be a nutritionist.

Diagnosis:

After thorough examination on her behavior, Nancy's actions had nothing to do with an attitude problem. In fact, it was all due to the type of food they had been feeding her.

Treatment:

Because she ate a lot of sweets, I decided to recommend the removal of milk and juices from her diet. I first imposed a zero sugar and carbohydrates diet on Nancy. I then added protein to the child's regimen and replaced cereals and milk with eggs for breakfast.

I even recommended a haircut. Nancy's waist-long hair was cut because it actually consumes a lot of nutrients that she could not afford to lose.

Result:

After three days undergoing the changes, Nancy basically became an entirely new person. She had better attitude at home with no more temper issues, which surprised her parents. She even improved in her studies so much so that she was near the top of her class with a grade card full of A's and B's. Her confidence was also boosted because of this achievement.

Analysis:

The foods we eat highly affect bodily processes that we never thought were connected to our gut. There are certain foods that cause utter chaos in the body. Some of these cause intestinal permeability or the so-called leaky gut. When a person has this condition, the cells in the intestines that are supposedly tightly-joined unravel, resulting in a leak of the proteins and other macromolecules into the bloodstream.

And because they haven't been transformed into energy yet, these proteins are attacked by the body's immune system, considering them foreign objects that have no business being in the blood. This often leads to autoimmune disorder.

In Nancy's case, her gut was not able to respond appropriately to the large amount of sugars that entered her body. And because it was not allowed ample time—about 72 hours—to repair itself, the gut became leaky and had so many issues that it failed to break down proteins into amino acids and other nutrients, which are supposed to be transmitted into the other parts of the body, including the brain.

As a big proponent of diet as a cure to ADD, schools should not immediately refer students to doctors who give medications to children who show signs of the disorder but instead have a nutritionist look into their diet to rule out any issues in their gut that can greatly affects their mental capabilities.

Having an unhealthy gut causes a ripple of medical conditions that could have been prevented using a simple but regular medical detox.

Nutrition has a close relationship with health. Studies have proven that people who eat whole foods rich in essential nutrients are likely to enjoy good health, longer life and diminished risks of many diseases. Eating nutritious foods also helps to maintain a normal body weight. Before getting into the nutritional regimen, I recommend getting a test for nutritional deficiencies. The test will tell which aspect of your health we need to focus on.

Blood test for nutritional deficiencies

Vitamins are very important to everyone. Decreased levels of these essentials nutrients can lead to life threatening conditions and vigorously limit the body's strength to fight off certain infections and diseases. Vitamin and nutrition blood tests can reveal mineral, iron, calcium, gluten, and other deficiencies.

A comprehensive test is important in letting you know which vitamins are lacking in your body and which you are not getting sufficient amounts through natural sources. These tests are available to measure the levels of micronutrients present in your body. It is not enough just to take supplements, it is also important to know how much and which one you should consider taking to balance the levels in your body.

Some common signs of nutrient deficiency

A nutrient deficiency can sometimes be tricky. Unless you are gravely deficient for some time, you may not notice any symptoms, which would lead you to believe that your body is assimilating all that your body needs. Commonly, nutrient deficiencies can cause symptoms, which can be mild or severe. Some common symptoms of micronutrient deficiencies include:

1. **Piercing, tingling or numbness in your limbs.** This can be a sign of Vitamin B deficiency, particularly Folate, B12 and B6. This greatly affects the peripheral nerves and can be a combination of depression, anxiety, fatigue, anemia and hormonal imbalances.

2. **White or Red acne-like bumps on the thighs, arms, cheeks and buttocks.** This can be a symptom of Vitamin A and D deficiency, or essential fatty acids like Omega 3s.

3. **Muscle cramps.** Muscle cramps is a common symptom of Magnesium, Calcium and Potassium deficiency. If certain parts of your body like your

toes, leg muscles, arches of your feet, or calves frequently experiences this, then it is a deficiency in those essential nutrients.

4. **Red scaly rash on the face and hair loss.** This can be a Vitamin B7 deficiency. The body utilizes the vitamin, biotin, in metabolizing fats, amino acids and carbohydrates, but it is also needed to strengthen hair and nails.

5. **Crack in the corner of the mouth.** This is a common sign that you are body is lacking the nutrients Iron, Zinc, Vitamins B12, Niacin and Riboflavin. The absorption of iron needs the aid of Vitamin C so it is also a must to take in Vitamin C to facilitate the absorption of the body of the mineral.

Get a thyroid test

The thyroid gland creates hormones that are important for normal metabolism. A thyroid function test is a sequence of blood tests used to measure how the thyroid gland is working. The test includes T3, T4 and TSH. These series of tests can describe whether the thyroid produces normal, overactive or underactive production of hormones in the blood.

186

The thyroid is a small gland found in the lower front part of your neck. It is important in regulating most of the body's processes including metabolism, energy production and overall mood. The thyroid produces two main hormones, the triiodothyronine (T3) and thyroxine (T4).

If the thyroid does not produce enough of these hormones, they eventually lead to common symptoms such as weight gain, depression and lack of energy. This is what is what is known as hypothyroidism.

If the thyroid creates too much hormones, there can be weight loss, elevation towards anxiety, a sense of being high and tremors. This is what is called as hyperthyroidism.

Commonly, you would ask your doctor for a thyroid test such as a T4 or a Thyroid-Stimulating Hormone (TSH) test. If the results of these tests come back anomalous, I would suggest further testing to pinpoint the main reason for the problem. This is usually done before we start with the program.

Understanding the test results

The triiodothyronine or T3 and thyroxine T4 are systemic within the body. The T4 tests and TSH test are the most common thyroid function test and are oftentimes ordered together.

A high level of T4 in the blood would indicate an overactive thyroid. Common symptoms experienced would include unexpected weight loss, tremors, diarrhea, and anxiety. This means that you have hyperthyroidism.

The TSH test is done to measure the level of thyroid-stimulating hormone in the blood, normal units are between point four to four mIU/L in the blood. One sign of hypothyroidism is when you have a TSH level of above two mIU/L, there is a great risk for you to advancing to hypothyroidism. The common symptoms of this is weight gain, depression, fatigue and frailness of fingernails and brittleness of hair.

The T3 test is administered to check the level of triiodothyronine in the blood. It is usually done if the T4 test and TSH test suggest abnormal activity. A T3 test is done if you are showing symptoms of an overactive or underactive thyroid gland. An abnormally high level of triiodothyronine found in the blood commonly leads to a condition called Grave's disease, an autoimmune disease often associated with hyperthyroidism.

The T3 Resin Uptake or T3RU, is a blood test used to measure the levels of proteins that carry thyroid hormone in the blood. A common indication of your T3 levels being high, is that these binding hormones are low. A high level of T3RU is a common indication that there may be an existing problem with the kidney or the body may not be getting enough protein. Low levels of T3RU is often due to pregnancy, obesity, hormone replacement therapy or eating estrogen-rich foods.

Nutrients that may help the thyroid

The thyroid gland uses distinct vitamins and minerals to properly do its job. Knowing this it is best to know which nutrients are out of balance. This way, we are able to adjust food intake and provide supplementation. There are key nutrients that are beneficial in promoting a healthy thyroid. Some of them are:

1. Iodine. This is the most significant trace mineral needed by the thyroid for it to function properly. Without iodine, the thyroid will not have the fundamental building blocks needed to create its hormones.
2. Triiodothyronine (T3) and Thyroxine (T4), are the most important and active iodine containing hormones in our body.

3. Selenium. Selenium is crucial to our thyroid for several reasons. Selenium-holding enzymes help defend our thyroid gland when we experience stress. It works by flushing out chemical and oxidative agents from our body. Selenium-based proteins support in regulating hormone synthesis and modifying T4 into the more usable T3. These

proteins and enzymes helps regulate the proper amount of thyroid hormones in our body including tissues, the blood and vital organs such as the kidneys, liver and the brain. Selenium also regulates metabolism and reuse of stored iodine.

4. Zinc, Iron and Copper. These three trace metals are important to thyroid function because they help adjust its function. A flat level of zinc can cause T3, T4, and TSH to become low. It has been shown that hyperthyroidism and hypothyroidism can deplete the body's zinc level which leads to lowered thyroid hormones. Lack of iron also reduces the thyroid's function. Copper helps in the production of TSH and management of T4 creation.

5. Vitamin B and Antioxidants. B Vitamins are optimal for thyroid health. These vitamins help to regulate the utilization of iodine at a cellular level. Antioxidants also aid the thyroid in diminishing the effects of oxidative stress. Antioxidants act as a barrier before the thyroid gets damaged due to oxidative stress.

Changes in the body and organs affected by thyroid problems

Thyroid glands. Deterioration of the thyroid gland greatly affects the body's metabolism. The end effect of this can be seen with weight easily gained or lost. An autoimmune disorder, Hashimoto's disease can cause both weight gain and loss depending on the phase of autoimmune deterioration of the thyroid gland.

Nervous System (CNS). The central nervous system can be hugely affected by a thyroid problem. The nervous system can either react too little or too much to the production of thyroid hormone. Poor hormone production can cause mental lethargy while too many hormones bring about nervousness and anxiety. Research and studies conducted have also linked hypothyroidism and Hashimoto's disease to the brain's quick degeneration and advancement of diseases like Parkinson's, Huntington's and Alzheimer's.

Digestive System. Chronic constipation is linked to hypothyroidism while frequent bowel movement is associated with hyperthyroidism. These symptoms are somewhat due to altered metabolism but can also be related to defective digestion starting in the stomach. Hypothyroidism can lessen the production of stomach acid inherent to the hormone, gastrin. When the stomach produces too little gastrin, decreased food digestion, intestinal inflammation and heartburn can result due to lack of regular stomach acid level.

Cardiovascular System. Although it has minimal reaction on the cardiovascular system, the response of too little or too much thyroid hormones circulating in the blood has its inherent effects. Hyperthyroidism can cause faster heart rate with higher blood pressure and atrial fibrillation. Insomnia is usually linked with hyperthyroidism. Insomnia is also akin to the decreased amount of serotonin circulating in the blood that is also associated with gut issues and can be identified with thyroid problems.

Adrenal Glands.

Thyroid function has complex ties with adrenal health. Part of the functional treatment of thyroid problems involve the adrenal gland because of various reasons. Among them is that adrenal fatigue causes the thyroid receptors on cells to give up their sensitivity to thyroid hormones. Adrenal fatigue can also cut back on the adaptability of the immune system walls in the gut, blood, lungs and brain barriers. It also obstructs the absorption of thyroid hormones in the cells. Adrenal fatigue also disturbs the give and take connection between the pituitary gland and hypothalamus with the thyroid gland.

Some common signs of a thyroid problem

As with other diseases, there are tell-tale signs that you may have a problem with your thyroid. All the symptoms listed below are indication of the problem and you may not have all of them.

192

1. **Fatigue and exhaustion after eight hours of sleep.** Feeling drained and exhausted when you wake up after getting eight hours of sleep is one symptom. This is one indication that you may have hypothyroidism. Hyperthyroidism on the other hand, leaves you restless at night and keeps you exhausted during the day.

2. **Weight gain or the inefficiency to lose weight.** Undefined weight issues and changes can both be a hint of hypothyroidism or hyperthyroidism. Being on a constant dietary regimen and not seeing any changes or even gaining more than what you are working on is a sign of hypothyroidism. If you are losing weight fast, then that is a sign of hyperthyroidism. Consult your doctor immediately.

3. **Mood swings, depression and anxiety.** Mood swings, depression and anxiety or any sudden outbreak of panic disorder is a symptom of a thyroid issue. Hypothyroidism is most often related to depression. Hyperthyroidism is typically associated with panic attacks, anxiety, and bipolar disease.

4. **Hormonal imbalances, irregular menstrual periods and infertility.** Women who have hypothyroidism are prone to miscarriages and infertility. They have a heavier, painful and more frequent period. Those with hyperthyroidism suffer from shorter and infrequent menstruation or even

the total arrest of menstrual period.

5. **Muscle and joint pains, tendonitis, Carpal Tunnel Syndrome.** People with hypothyroidism can experience muscle pains and aches specifically in the arms and legs. They also have a greater risk of developing Carpal Tunnel Syndrome, a painful condition wherein there is a compression of the major nerve in the carpal bones.

6. **Hair loss and skin changes.** The hair and nails are body parts susceptible to thyroid conditions. Hair loss, in particular is often linked to thyroid problems. People with hypothyroidism experience having coarse, brittle, and dry hair which falls off easily. Their skin becomes thick, dry and scaly. With hyperthyroidism, severe hair loss can often develop and the skin can develop irritations and can be sensitive and delicate. Skin rashes can also appear on the shins called thyroid dermopathy or pretibial myxedema.

7. **Constipation, diarrhea and bowel problems.** Constant severe constipation that does not subside despite medications is commonly linked to hypothyroidism while diarrhea, and irritable bowel syndrome or IBS is common with hyperthyroidism.

8. **High cholesterol levels despite medications.** High levels of cholesterol in the blood despite medications and diet can be a sign of

194

hypothyroidism. While having low cholesterol levels may be a symptom of hyperthyroidism.

9. **Neck swelling and discomfort, goiter and hoarseness.** An evident enlargement and discomfort in the neck, difficulty swallowing and a raspy voice is a tell-tale sign of the disease. Developing a goiter can either be a sign of hypothyroidism or hyperthyroidism.

10. **Family history of thyroid problems.** Having a history in the family of thyroid problems greatly increases your risk of contracting one. Be aware of autoimmune diseases such as rheumatoid arthritis in the family as these increases your risk of getting autoimmune thyroid problems like Grave's or Hashimoto's disease.

How a change in metabolism affect thyroid function?

Detoxification for the thyroid

Detoxification can be a process not only to improve the function of the thyroid but it can also be beneficial to overall health. The process dispels and cleans out many of the toxins, xenohormones and other impurities in the body and leaves a feeling of good health.

Detoxifying the thyroid starts with the gut and the liver. Those two systems have a direct link to the overall health of the thyroid. Studies have shown that people who have a problem with their thyroid usually have multiple digestive issues and a slacking liver.

You may know you have digestive issues when you experience constipation, loose stool, diarrhea, bloating, acid reflux, and gas. You may also crave for foods rich in sugar and starches and feel incomplete without them. You may also know you have a digestive problem if you have been on medication for a long period of time in the past and in most serious cases, you have irritable bowel syndrome, Celiac or Crohn's disease.

The Gut-Liver-Thyroid connection has an important role in the regulation of thyroid hormones.

We must also consider our immune system. Almost 90% of thyroid problems are autoimmune problems. If you are suffering from hypothyroidism, chances are you have Hashimoto's disease. What an autoimmune disease means is that your immune system is responding differently by slowly destroying your thyroid. As a consequence of the immune system's actions, the thyroid gland slows down and is the reason why you tend to feel bad.

One common trait of people with thyroid problems the absorption of nutrients. The gut is primarily responsible for this function. Almost all people with thyroid disease are deficient in essential vitamins like Vitamin D, B12 and minerals like selenium and iron among others. This is because their gut is not absorbing most of the nutrients and is in a state of what is known as dysbiosis, a common state where there is a microbial imbalance in the body.

The gut is also known as the second brain because there are more neurotransmitters located in the gut than in the brain. Serotonin, or the happy hormone is largely produced in the gut not in the brain. This is why when we experience digestive problems, we often feel somber or depressed because the gut is not generating serotonin adequately.

What most thyroid patients do not recognize is that the thyroid creates T4 which is an inactive hormone. T4 needs to be changed and converted to T3 in the liver and in the gut so it can turn on energy and metabolism. If the liver functions slowly, conversion of the hormone can be slow and ineffective.

Simple exercises that are beneficial to thyroid health

There are some exercises in which the thyroid has an indirect benefit. Simple exercises that you can do at home or in the office and that elevates your heart rate have an effect not only on your whole body but on the thyroid as well. Three minutes a day for starting an exercise regime would greatly help to keep the body active and strengthen hormone production. Some of these exercises are in the form that can exercise major muscles in the body. They are:

Squats and lunges - Squats help exhaust and build muscles in the legs including the quadriceps, calves and hamstrings. Doing squats also generates the release of testosterone and growth hormones in the body which are important for building muscle mass.

Pushing or dumbbell exercises - Pushing exercises or a simple push-up can strengthen your upper muscles. Doing these exercises with or without equipment as long as the heart rate is elevated helps regulate the functions of the systems in your body.

Lat pulldown or pull ups. Lat pulldowns do not require much agility. It is a multi-joint exercise that includes movement at the elbows, shoulders and scapula. Other parts of the body such as the biceps, rhomboids and traps are also involved during a pulldown exercise.

Concluding Words

The thyroid gland plays a huge role in every stage of our life. From infancy to old age, having a healthy and functioning thyroid will keep us away from infections and life threatening diseases. It acts as the engine that powers up the immune system, metabolism, muscle and skeletal growth, and reproductive development. Without the thyroid, your brain, liver, heart, and kidneys will never function properly.

Just in the U.S., there are over 30 million Americans who are suffering from thyroid problems and half of them remain undiagnosed. Of the sexes, women are eight times more at risk to this health issue than men. Though manageable, undiagnosed thyroid problems can lead to thyroid cancer, diabetes, infertility, miscarriage, and cardiovascular diseases. Thus, it is important to have your thyroid checked at least once to twice a year to maintain your thyroid's health and avoid long term issues.

If you are having problems losing weight and are experiencing a few or most of the symptoms discussed in this book, immediately visit an endocrinologist and have your neck checked for further evaluation of your health condition. Getting to the root of the problem is the easiest way to find a solution and address the issue effectively. The problem may not be your physical activity or how many calories you have burned throughout your weight loss program. The problem could be much deeper.

And of course, prevention is better than cure. You might not have thyroid problems right now, but this is not an excuse to neglect your thyroid's health. Follow a regulated and holistic lifestyle. And by holistic, we mean that you become wise in your food choices, your decisions in life, and your daily activities. Do not abuse your body to the point where it starts to become imbalanced and malfunctioned. The body, by nature, knows how to heal itself. However, when you begin to abuse your body, its natural rhythm begins to decline, opening itself to infections and diseases.

Bring back your body's natural balance by leading a life wherein you begin to respect its capacity and limitation. You take care of your mind by practicing yoga and meditation, being outdoors, working on your passion, and praying.

And when your body starts to regain its rhythm, balance, and vitality, losing weight and improving your overall health will easily follow.